Bike Paths

OF MASSACHUSETTS

A Guide to Rail-Trails
& Other Car-Free Places

STUART JOHNSTONE

Active Publications
P.O. Box 1037
Concord, MA 01742

Published by: Active Publications
P.O. Box 1037
Concord, MA 01742-1037

Printed in the United States of America

Publisher's Cataloging in Publication Data

Johnstone, Stuart A.
Bike Paths of Massachusetts: A Guide to Rail-Trails &
Other Car-Free Places / by Stuart A. Johnstone; photographs by
the author.
ISBN 978-0-692-90339-1
1. Bicycle touring - Massachusetts - Guidebooks
2. Massachusetts - Description and travel

Dedicated

to active transportation and recreation,
and to the people and places that inspire it.

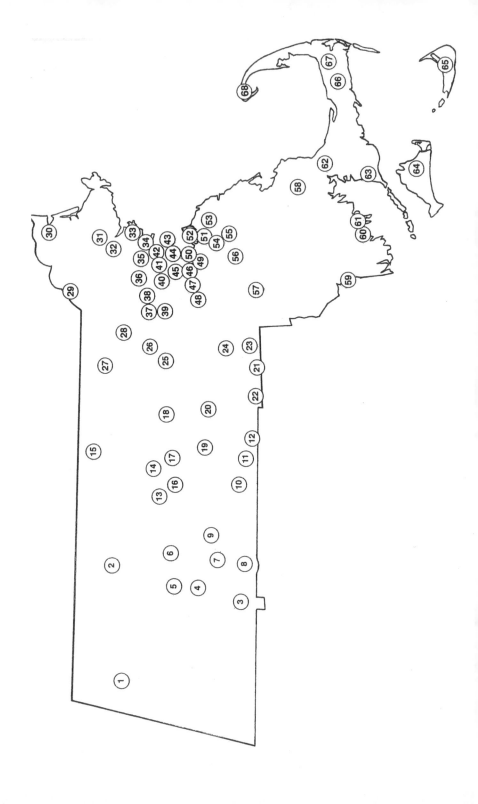

Contents

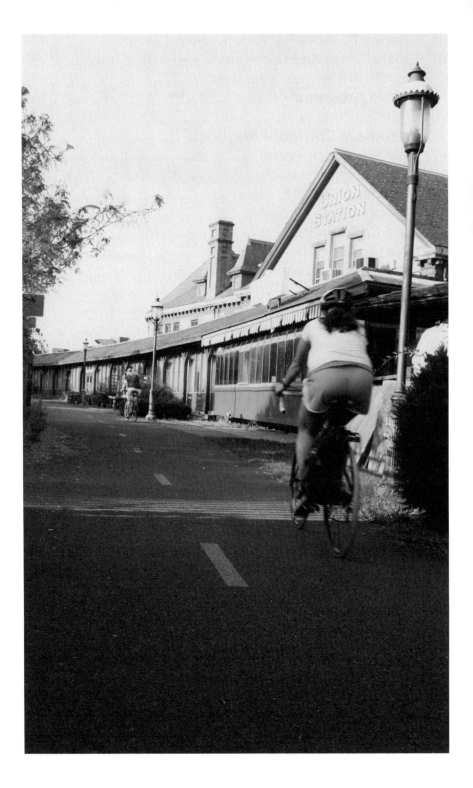

Introduction

Bike paths make important connections. Not only do they join places with safe, car-free transportation and recreation but they also connect people to communities in subtle, friendly ways that roads can seldom match. They also connect families with nature, commuters with fitness, the environmental health of an area with its economic vitality, and the future with the past. Most importantly, bike paths and other forms of bike/pedestrian infrastructure lead us to live more sustainably as they inspire people of all ages and abilities to leave their cars behind and enjoy the freedom and other benefits of active transportation. Traveling a trail brings people to a better place and, not coincidently, gives them the chance to say hello to others along the way.

Human-powered mobility has a bright future in Massachusetts as the diverse and growing array of prepared-surface trails, both paved and unpaved, now totals over 600 miles and connects more communities than ever. New bike paths are being constructed, existing paths are being lengthened, and many are being joined in networks toward the vision of a state connected by multi-use trails. Ranging from urban to rural, the options include flat, easy rail-trails as well as free-flowing paths through a variety of landscapes in state parks and other public lands. The most popular options attract steady streams of human-powered traffic but others venture into remote areas with solitude.

Bike Paths of Massachusetts has been written from the bicyclist's perspective but will also appeal to walkers and other human-powered travelers. An important objective of the book is to communicate rules and regulations, standards of trail etiquette, and safety features for the trails since the locations vary widely and each has its own set of conditions. Set yourself in motion and enjoy your explorations!

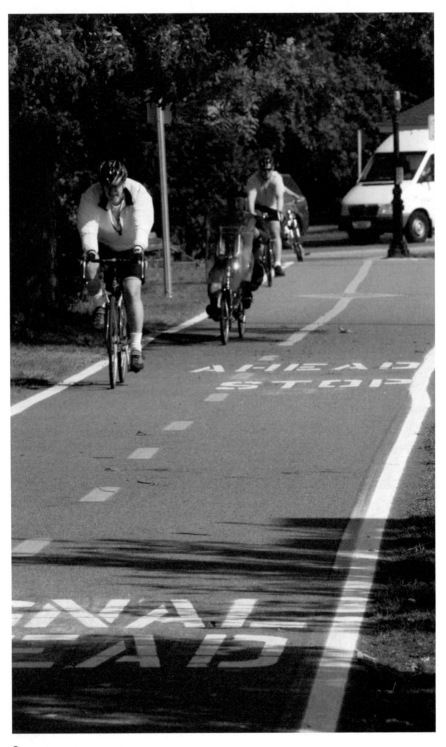

Rules of the Bike Path

1. **Keep to the right.** Most bike paths have two-way traffic so stay on the right side to allow safe passage. Remember that others might need to pass you.
2. **Pass on the left after signaling audibly.** Make verbal contact (*"On your left..."*) or signal with a bell to avoid startling the slower traveler. Look both ahead and behind before passing.
3. **Yield to pedestrians and horseback riders.** Bicyclists and in-line skaters are expected to yield to slower travelers.
4. **Stop at road crossings and look both ways.** Drivers will not always be aware of bike path crossings so assume that they do not see you.
5. **Stay alert and be predictable.** Anticipate the actions of others and let them anticipate yours by avoiding sudden changes in movement. Use extra caution when children and pets are present.
6. **Do not block the bike path when stopped.** Step off the surface to allow others to pass unimpeded.

   Massachusetts state law requires that bicyclists aged 16 and under wear approved helmets. All ages should be aware that serious injuries are possible on bike paths and that the risk of accidents increases in the presence of children, pets, groups of people, and intersections. Bicyclists, because they can travel relatively quickly and quietly, present additional risk for collisions.

   Bike paths are not meant for speed. Cyclists planning on riding fast should either use roads or take care in choosing an appropriate place and time.

   Noise and litter have a negative impact for other bike path users and for abutting property owners. Respect the

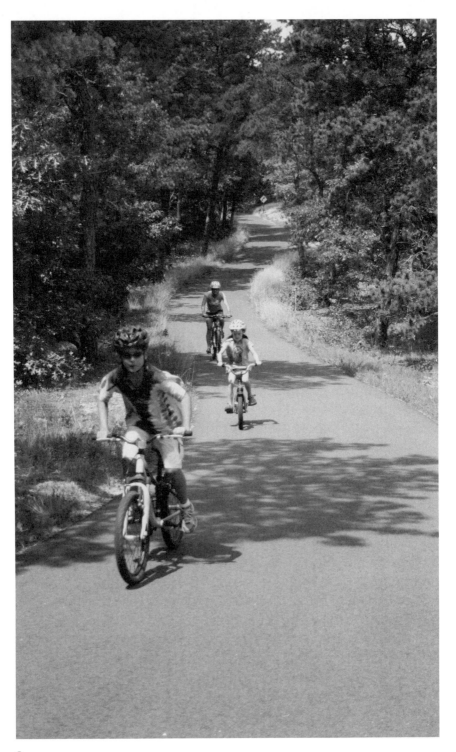

environment of the trail so that others can also enjoy it.

Hunting occurs near bike paths in some areas. The most active hunting period is deer season in the late fall, when trail users are encouraged to wear an article of "blaze orange" clothing. Hunting is prohibited by state law on Sundays.

Pet owners should be aware of local leash laws and rules regarding animal wastes. Owners are required to remove their pets' wastes at most trails.

When parking, avoid leaving valuables in your car, even if it is locked. Park at designated locations and be careful not to block trailhead gates because work crews and emergency vehicles always need access.

Planning Your Trip

Be prepared! Getting lost, underestimating trip length or difficulty, and overestimating physical capabilities can bring undesireable consequences especially in remote areas. A weather change or equipment failure can ruin an otherwise wonderful time. Be ready for unwanted surprises by planning ahead and bringing some useful items.

Drinking water is one of the most essential things to remember, especially in summer. It is easy to become dehydrated while exercising so carry a water bottle or two on the bike or on your body and start drinking before you get thirsty. Longer tours require greater amounts.

Even if you are not planning a picnic, bring something to eat on longer excursions in case your body runs low on energy. A snack can give an important boost both physically and psychologically.

If you are unsure of the trails that you plan to explore, carry a map and keep track of the features that you pass such as road intersections, bridges, and bodies of water. Track mileage using a cyclometer which mounts on the handlebars and displays distance, time, speed, and other information to assist with navigating.

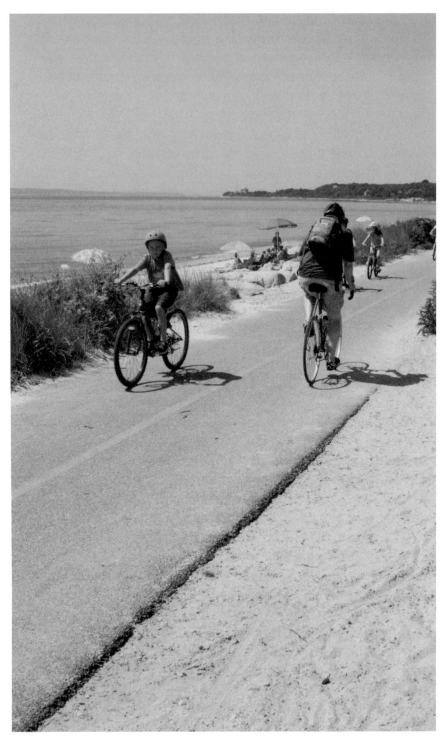

Bicyclists should consider bringing tools for simple repairs. Since many of the bike paths described in this book reach isolated places, riders will have an important advantage in being able to fix a flat tire or repair a simple mechanical problem when necessary. Most helpful will be a pump, which can be fitted to the bike frame, and either a spare inner tube or patch kit to seal inner tube leaks. An adjustable wrench and screwdriver can also be helpful. If you are not capable of making general repairs and are not self-sufficient with tools when venturing into remote areas, it is wise to ride with others who are.

Other useful items include bug repellent during spring and summer, extra clothing to suit possible weather changes, and first aid supplies. These items add minimal weight relative to their potential benefits.

For safety, ride with a companion and leave word of your planned route with a responsible person.

What to Wear

If you are traveling on wheels, the most important item is a bike helmet. Light and comfortable to wear, it should be worn by all ages as valuable protection from the hazards encountered along a trail. **Massachusetts state law requires bike helmets for ages 16 and under**. Since three quarters of all bicycle-related deaths result from head injuries, wearing a helmet is a healthy habit regardless of age. In-line skaters are encouraged to also wear knee, elbow, and wrist protection.

Wear comfortable clothing and dress in layers to allow adjustments for temerature and also to suit possible weather changes.

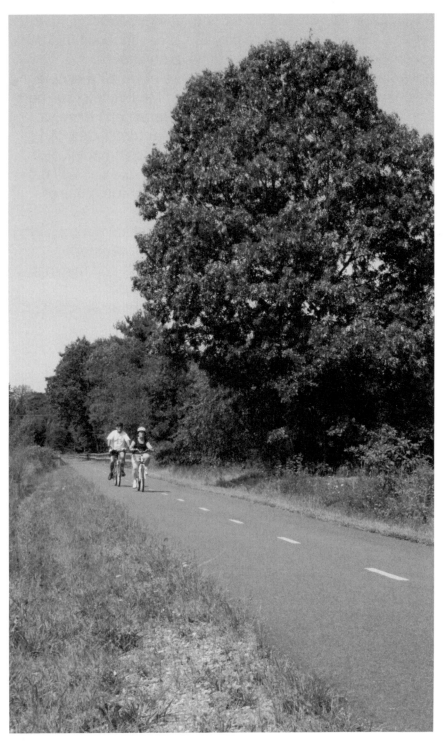

About This Guidebook

   Bike Paths of Massachusetts is meant to be a starting point, a means for people to discover places for themselves. It has been written to prepare readers with rules, trail descriptions, and suggested destinations so that they can better enjoy their explorations. Narrated directions should be recognized as only one of perhaps several ways to tour an area.

   Maps are provided to give a general view of trail networks and natural features. Note that the map scale for each area varies widely so plan your distances and courses carefully. The names of trails, roads, and surrounding landmarks appear with boldface type in the text for quick referencing. Only the major parking areas are designated on maps so smaller spots might also exist.

   Background information includes pieces of local history for each bike path. Most of the railroad history regarding rail-trails originates from *The Rail Lines of Southern New England* (1995, Branch Line Press, ISBN 0-942147-02-2), by Ronald Karr.

   Practical information accompanies each description. This includes the locations of toilet facilities when present and sources of additional information. Driving directions originate from nearby highways and will be most helpful when used together with a road map.

   Since improvements to the region's bike paths are ongoing, be aware that in some cases the length, surface, and other amenities of a trail might be better than they are described in this book.

Get involved!

   Plenty of bike path projects would benefit from your help. Volunteer your time and/or money for the benefit of a favorite or a future trail in your area and be part of the progress!

1

Ashuwillticook Rail-Trail

Lanesborough-Adams

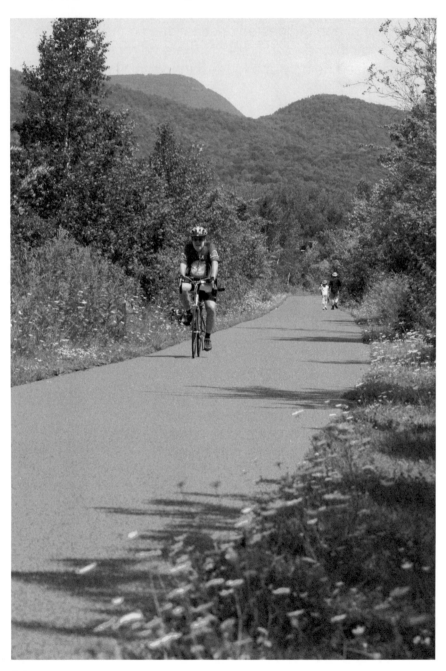

LENGTH: 12.1 miles
SURFACE: paved
TERRAIN: slight slopes

One of Massachusetts' most scenic rail-trails, the 3-town Ashuwillticook offers a welcomingly steady course through the Berkshires with mountain, lake, and river views.

RULES & SAFETY:
• Bicyclists should yield to pedestrians.
• Keep to the right, pass on the left, and alert others (*"On your left..."*) when approaching from behind.
• Be especially cautious in the presence of children and pets since their movements can be unpredictable.
• Step off the trail when stopped to allow others to pass.
• Stop at road intersections and assume that drivers do not see you. Crosswalk signals exist at some intersections.
• Dogs must be leashed and their wastes removed.

ORIENTATION:
The trail parallels Rte. 8 for its entire length with appealing scenery in each of the towns of Lanesborough, Cheshire, and Adams. The southern end (Lanesborough) has the highest elevation and the northern end (Adams) has the lowest, but the slope is only noticeable along 2.5 miles in Adams. Be aware that the southernmost trailhead at Berkshire Mall Rd. is often full on fairweather weekends.

TRAIL DESCRIPTION:
Beginning in Lanesborough at **Berkshire Mall Rd.**, the Ashuwillticook heads north curving through wetlands for the first mile to **Berkshire Pond** where water views open the scenery. After crossing **Old State Rd.** (1.7 miles), the Cheshire town line, and **Nobody's Rd.** (2.4 miles), the trail follows 2.5 miles of shoreline at 3-basin **Cheshire Reservoir** where longer views spread to surrounding Berkshire hills. A trailhead at **Farnams St.** (3.7 miles) offers toilets and picnicking at the reservoir's midpoint.

The trail intersects **Rte. 8** (5.2 miles) at a signaled crosswalk near the center of **Cheshire** and follows the

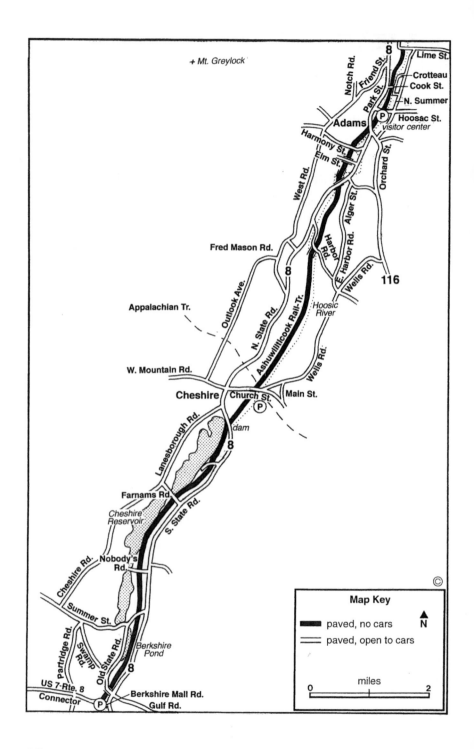

+ *Mt. Greylock*

Notch Rd.

Friend St.

8

Lime St.

Crotteau

Cook St.

Park St.

N. Summer

Adams

Ⓟ

Hoosac St.

visitor center

Harmony St.

Elm St.

West Rd.

Alger St.

Orchard St.

Fred Mason Rd.

Harbor Rd.

E. Harbor Rd.

Wells Rd.

116

8

Outlook Ave.

Appalachian Tr.

N. State Rd.

Ashuwillticook Rail-Tr.

Hoosic River

W. Mountain Rd.

Wells Rd.

Cheshire

Church St.

Main St.

Ⓟ

dam

8

Lanesborough Rd.

S. State Rd.

Farnams Rd.

Cheshire Reservoir

Cheshire Rd.

Nobody's Rd.

Summer St.

Partridge Rd.

Swamp Rd.

Old State Rd.

Berkshire Pond

8

US 7-Rte. 8

Connector

Ⓟ

Berkshire Mall Rd.

Gulf Rd.

©

Map Key

▲
N

paved, no cars

paved, open to cars

miles

0   2

16

Hoosic River for the next three quarters of a mile. After passing the **Church St.** trailhead (5.9 miles) and the **Appalachian Tr.**, the rail-trail enjoys quiet, natural scenery as it traverses 2 miles of open wetland with distant views.

Returning to woods, it then crosses a bridge over the Hoosic at **Harbor Rd.** (8.3 miles), named for its history along the Underground Railroad, and descends with a noticeable slope on a shelf cut into a tight valley. Bridges allow it to pass under Rte. 8 (9.5 miles), over the river, and under **Elm St.** After intersecting **Harmony St.** (10.2 miles) at a playing field, the trail follows the riverbank to a signaled crosswalk at **Park St./Rte. 8** in downtown **Adams** (10.6 miles), passes the former train station, and reaches the **Adams Visitor Center** (10.9 miles) where toilets and parking are available.

North of the visitor center and **Hoosac St.** (10.9 miles) the trail's newest leg continues downstream intersecting **Cook St.** (11.4 miles) and then veering off the rail bed along the riverbank to the current endpoint at **Lime St.** (12.1 miles), named for a limestone quarry visible nearby.

BACKGROUND:

This route was created in 1845 as the Pittsfield & North Adams Railroad and served as a secondary line between other railroads until 1990. After a successful effort to preserve the right of way, construction of the trail's first section was completed in 2001, the second in 2003, and a 1.2-mile northern extension was made in 2017. Future extensions are planned for both ends of the trail.

Ashuwillticook is a Native American name meaning *"at the pleasant river in between the hills."*

DRIVING DIRECTIONS:

• **Berkshire Mall Rd. from Rte. 9:** Follow Rte. 8 north for 1.5 miles, then turn left on Berkshire Mall Rd.

• **Adams trailhead from Rte. 2:** Follow Rte. 8 south for 5.5 miles, turn left on Hoosac St., then right on Depot St. Park at the Adams Visitor Center immediately on the left.

TOILETS:

Berkshire Mall Rd., Farnams St., Adams Visitor Center

ADDITIONAL INFORMATION:

Dept. of Conservation & Recreation, mass.gov/dcr
Berkshire Bike Path Council, www.berkshirebikepath.com

2 Canalside Trail
Montague-Deerfield

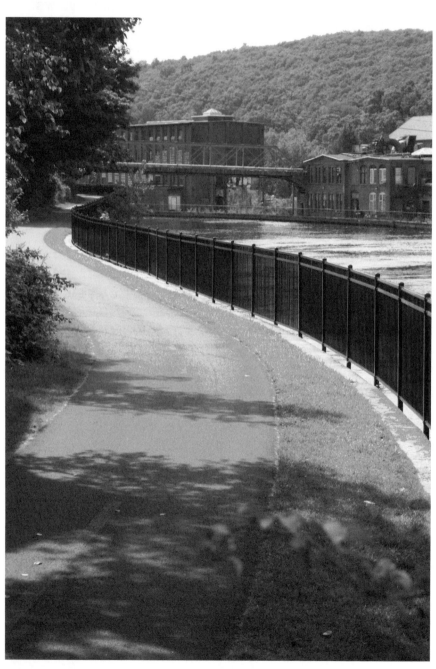

LENGTH: 3.6 miles (including 0.3-mile on-road section)
SURFACE: paved
TERRAIN: small slopes

This ride along the Connecticut River offers a variety of sights including a large dam and falls, a canal and hydro-electric facility, old factory buildings, peaceful woods, and a long trestle bridge spanning the flow.

RULES & SAFETY:
- Bicyclists should yield to pedestrians.
- Keep to the right, pass on the left, and alert others (*"On your left..."*) when approaching from behind.
- Use extra caution in the presence of children and pets since their movements can be unpredictable.
- Step off the trail when stopped so others can pass.
- Dogs must be leashed and their wastes removed.
- Swimming is prohibited in the canal.

ORIENTATION:
The trail exists in two sections separated by a marked, 0.3-mile on-road bike route along quiet streets with one busy road crossing. The 2.4-mile northern section has the most water views, limited shade, and the most usage while the 0.9-mile southern portion has woodsy surroundings and less usage. Trailheads access each part.

TRAIL DESCRIPTION:
Unity Park's playground, broad lawn, and waterfront view of the **Connecticut River** welcome visitors beside the village of **Turners Falls** (part of Montague) at the trail's northern end. Facing the water, turn left (west) and ride the paved trail under the **Avenue A** bridge, past an intersecting trail leading to the **Great Falls Discovery Center**, and downstream alongside a **canal.** Following a shelf on a slope lined by protective fencing, the trail curves southward (left) following the water's swift current past brick factory buildings on the way to **Turners Falls Rd.** (0.7 miles) and **11th St.** (1.2 miles), gradually leaving the village area for more open surroundings.

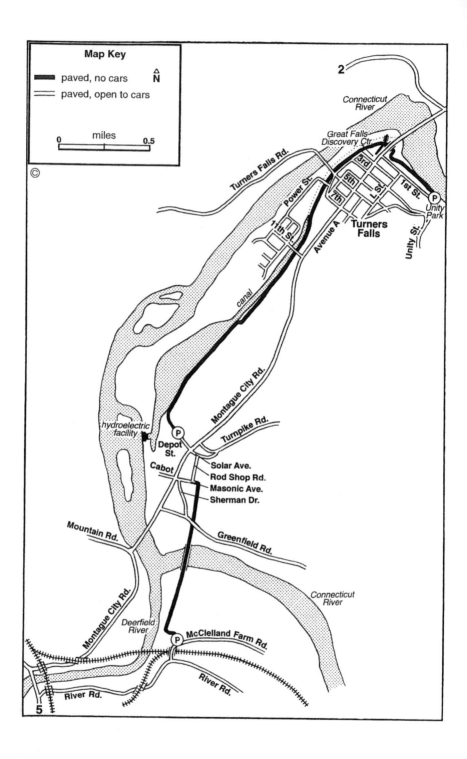

Map Key

— paved, no cars
= paved, open to cars

N

miles
0 — 0.5

©

2

Connecticut River

Great Falls
Discovery Ctr.

Turners Falls Rd.

Power St.

3rd
5th
7th
L St.
1st St.

Turners Falls

P
Unity Park

Unity St.

11th St.

Avenue A

canal

Montague City Rd.

Turnpike Rd.

hydroelectric facility

P
Depot St.

Cabot

Solar Ave.
Rod Shop Rd.
Masonic Ave.
Sherman Dr.

Mountain Rd.

Greenfield Rd.

Connecticut River

Montague City Rd.

Deerfield River

P **McClelland Farm Rd.**

River Rd.

River Rd.

5

It emerges on a dike built to contain the canal and straightens under a line of utility poles toward a **hydroelectric facility** before descending to a trailhead parking area at the end of **Depot Rd.** (2.4 miles).

Here a marked, 0.3-mile on-road bike route links the next section of trail. Continue along Depot Rd., cross **Montague City Rd.** (use caution), continue straight on **Solar Ave.**, turn right on **Rod Shop Rd.**, then left on **Masonic Ave.**

The trail resumes (2.7 miles) in woods heading south along a former rail bed that intersects **Greenfield Rd.** (3.0 miles) and emerges on a long trestle bridge spanning the Connecticut River. Nice views over the water include the confluence of the **Deerfield River** just upstream.

Returning to the cover of woods in neighboring Deerfield, the trail's final half-mile parallels a farm field then turns left off the rail bed and climbs a slope to a trailhead parking lot at **McClelland Farm Rd.** (3.6 miles).

BACKGROUND:

The Canalside Tr. utilizes a former Boston & Maine Railroad bed for much of its length. Opened in 1848, this rail line served Turners Falls' industries of paper, lumber, cotton, and cutlery, and operated until 1921 when its bridge over the Connecticut River was deemed unsafe. The nearby canal was originally built for navigating around the river's falls and was enlarged in 1915 for the generation of electricity. It continues to provide power for the region.

The Canalside Tr. was built in 2005 and extended southward a few years later, and is part of a future network of routes known as the Franklin County Bikeway.

DRIVING DIRECTIONS:

Unity Park from I-91: Take Exit 27 and follow Rte. 2 east for 2.8 miles, then turn right on Avenue A and cross the river to Turners Falls. Turn left on First St. and look for the parking lot ahead on the left where the road curves right.

McClellan Farm Rd. trailhead from I-91: Take Exit 26 and follow Rte. 2A east for 1 mile, then turn right on Rte. 5 south and continue for 1.4 miles. After crossing a bridge over the Deerfield River at the Deerfield town line, turn left on River Rd., drive for 0.9 miles, then turn left on McClellan Farm Rd. and park in the lot 0.1 miles ahead on the left.

3

Columbia Greenway
Southwick Rail-Trail
Farmington Canal Greenway

Westfield, MA-Farmington, CT

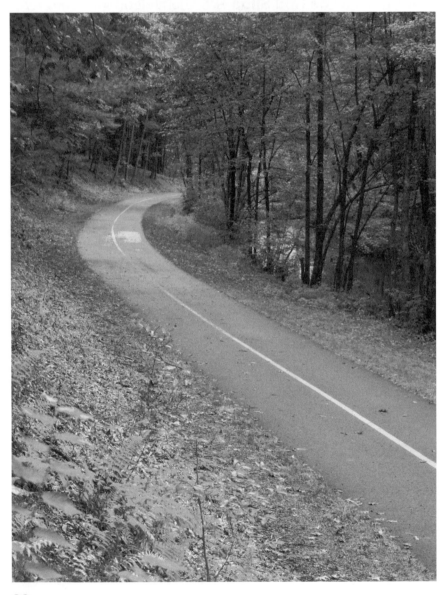

LENGTH: 30.9 miles
SURFACE: paved
TERRAIN: slight slopes, with hilly detours from the rail line

This grand rail-trail follows a historic route through eight towns in two states with a marathon of villages, forests, farmland, rivers, and remnants of the Farmington Canal.

RULES & SAFETY:
- Bicyclists should yield to pedestrians.
- Keep to the right, pass on the left, and alert others (*"On your left..."*) when approaching from behind.
- Be especially cautious in the presence of children and pets since their movements can be unpredictable.
- Groups should ride single file.
- Step off the trail when stopped so others can pass.
- Stop at road intersections and remember that drivers might not be aware of your presence.
- Respect nearby residents by keeping noise levels low.
- Pets must be leashed and their wastes removed.
- Watch for additional information posted at trailheads.

ORIENTATION:
The rail-trail assumes different names along its route. The Columbia Greenway refers to the Westfield, MA portion, the Southwick Rail-Trail refers to the Southwick, MA portion, and the Farmington Canal Heritage Tr. refers to the remaining distance in the Connecticut towns of Suffield, East Granby, Simsbury, Avon, and Farmington.

The trail is especially long so plan your trip length carefully. Scenery is good along the entire length but noticeably more rural along the northern half where woods and farmland allow greener surroundings and fewer road intersections. The map displays only the main trailheads and smaller parking areas exist at additional locations.

Elevation changes are minimal but cyclists will notice low points at river and stream bridges and higher points in between. Bigger slopes exist where the trail detours from the rail bed at the centers of Simsbury and Avon as well as other minor locations. Note that parts of the Avon detour utilize a marked, on-road route instead of separated pathway.

Crosswalks and signs are in place at road crossings and protective fencing borders the trail where necessary. Mileage markers along the trail in Connecticut originate at Red Oak Hill Rd. in Farmington. The presence of other amenities varies with location.

TRAIL DESCRIPTION:

Starting at the **Shaker Farms Country Club** trailhead parking lot, the **Columbia Greenway** runs in two directions. To the north, it extends for 2.1 miles to downtown **Westfield** with a scenic crossing of the **Little River** (0.7 miles) and surrounding farmland, a bridge over **E. Silver St.** (1.7 miles), and current endpoint at **Main St.** (2.1 miles). Follow Main St. a half-mile east (to the right) then turn left on **Meadow St.** to reach the **Westfield River Tr.**, a 1.5-mile pathway along a flood control dike beside the **Westfield River**.

Heading south, the trail extends for almost 29 miles and immediately enters Southwick as the **Southwick Rail Trail**. It climbs a small slope at **Sam West Rd.** (1.0 mile), cuts across a vast farm field before **Feeding Hills Rd./Rte. 57** (2.0 miles), and descends to **Depot St.** (2.8 miles) near **Southwick** center. After passing under **Point Grove Rd.** (3.2 miles), the trail gets only a hint of a view of nearby **Congamond Lake** at **Congamond Rd./Rte. 168** (5.1 miles).

Some of the best natural scenery lies along the next 6.5 miles. The trail passes a vast, open wetland on the right and joins the side of the original canal bed on the left before reaching the **state line** (6.3 miles) at Suffield, CT, where the **Farmington Canal Heritage Tr.** continues. After crossing a bridge over **Phelps Rd.** (6.7 miles), the trail cuts through an area of farm fields and hits the E. Granby town line on the way to **Copper Hill Rd.** (8.4 miles). It continues through an expanse of wooded wetlands for the next 1.5 miles to **Turkey Hills Rd./Rte. 20** (10.0 miles), intersects **Hartford Ave./Rte. 189** (11.0 miles), then crosses a curved bridge high above **Salmon Brook**.

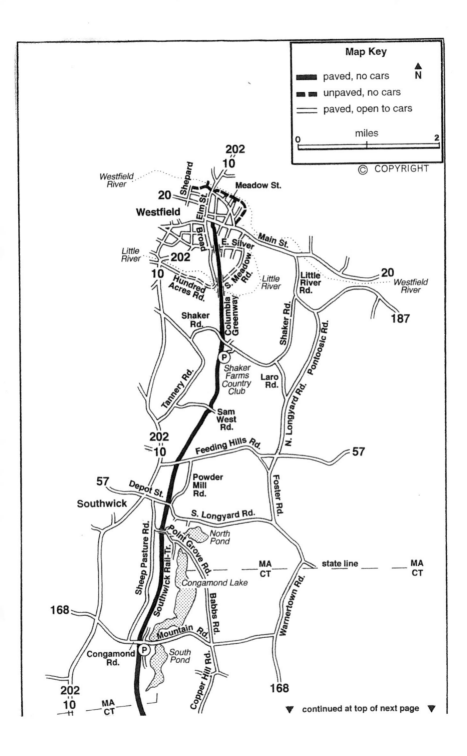

Map Key

▲ N

- ■■■ paved, no cars
- ■ ■ unpaved, no cars
- —— paved, open to cars

miles

0   2

© COPYRIGHT

202
10

Westfield River

Meadow St.

20

Shepard

Westfield

Elm St.

Broad

Main St.

E. Silver

Little River

202

10

Hundred Acres Rd.

S. Meadow Rd.

Little River

Little River Rd.

20

Westfield River

Shaker Rd.

Columbia Greenway

Shaker Rd.

187

P

Shaker Farms Country Club

Laro Rd.

Tannery Rd.

N. Longyard Rd.

Pontoosic Rd.

Sam West Rd.

202
10

Feeding Hills Rd.

57

57

Depot St.

Powder Mill Rd.

Foster Rd.

Southwick

S. Longyard Rd.

Sheep Pasture Rd.

Point Grove Rd.

Southwick Rail-Tr.

North Pond

MA
CT

state line

MA
CT

Congamond Lake

Warnertown Rd.

Babbs Rd.

168

Mountain Rd.

Congamond Rd.

P

South Pond

Copper Hill Rd.

168

202
10

MA
CT

▼ continued at top of next page ▼

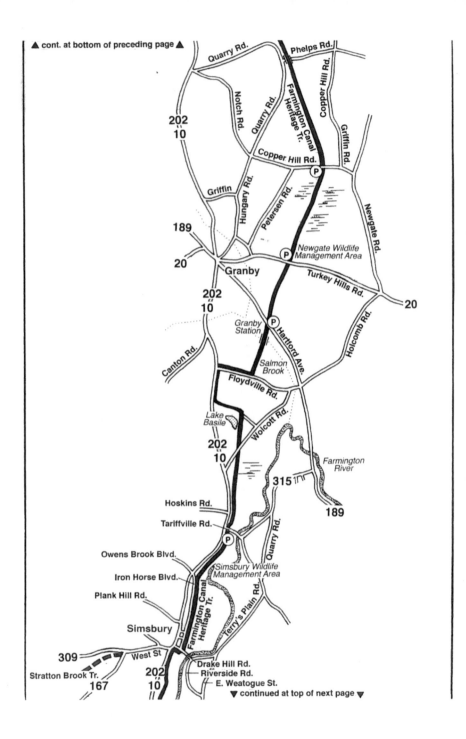

▲ cont. at bottom of preceding page ▲

Quarry Rd.

Phelps Rd.

Farmington Canal Heritage Tr.

Copper Hill Rd.

Notch Rd.

Quarry Rd.

Griffin Rd.

202
10

Copper Hill Rd.

P

Griffin

Hungary Rd.

Petersen Rd.

Newgate Rd.

189

20

P

Newgate Wildlife Management Area

Granby

Turkey Hills Rd.

20

202
10

Canton Rd.

Granby Station

P

Hartford Ave.

Holcomb Rd.

Salmon Brook

Floydville Rd.

Lake Basile

Wolcott Rd.

Farmington River

202
10

315

189

Hoskins Rd.

Tariffville Rd.

P

Quarry Rd.

Owens Brook Blvd.

Simsbury Wildlife Management Area

Iron Horse Blvd.

Terry's Plain Rd.

Plank Hill Rd.

Farmington Canal Heritage Tr.

Simsbury

309

West St

Stratton Brook Tr.

167

202
10

Drake Hill Rd.

Riverside Rd.

E. Weatogue St.

▼ continued at top of next page ▼

26

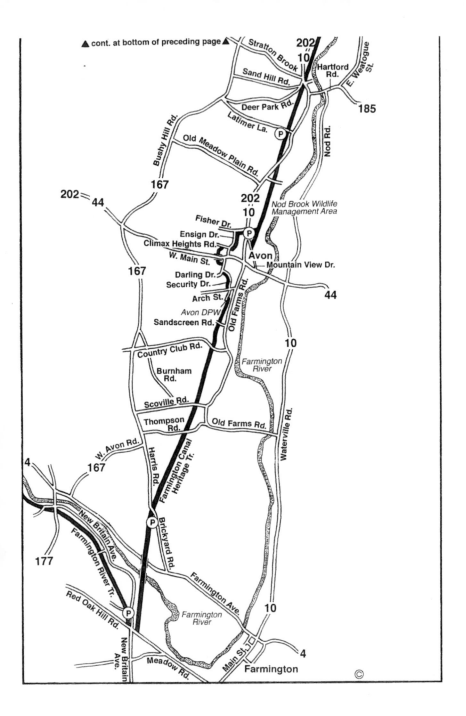

▲ cont. at bottom of preceding page ▲

Stratton Brook

202
10

Sand Hill Rd.

Hartford Rd.

E. Weatogue St.

Deer Park Rd.

185

Latimer La.

P

Old Meadow Plain Rd.

Bushy Hill Rd.

Nod Rd.

167

202
44

202
10

Nod Brook Wildlife Management Area

Fisher Dr.

Ensign Dr.

Climax Heights Rd.

P

W. Main St.

Avon

Mountain View Dr.

167

Darling Dr.

Security Dr.

Old Farms Rd.

Arch St.

44

Avon DPW

Sandscreen Rd.

Country Club Rd.

10

Burnham Rd.

Farmington River

Scoville Rd.

Thompson Rd.

Old Farms Rd.

Waterville Rd.

W. Avon Rd.

4

167

Harris Rd.

Farmington Canal Heritage Tr.

New Britain Ave.

P

Brickyard Rd.

177

Farmington River Tr.

Farmington Ave.

10

Red Oak Hill Rd.

P

Farmington River

4

New Britain Ave.

Main St.

Meadow Rd.

Farmington

©

27

A 1.7-mile detour off the rail bed begins at **Floydville Rd.** (11.8 miles). Circling agricultural fields, it turns right (west) beside the road and enters Granby, left beside **Rte. 10/202**, and left along a fence back to the rail line (13.5 miles).

The trail continues into Simsbury near **Lake Basile**, intersects **Wolcott Rd.** (14.0 miles), and passes behind a commercial area on Rte. 10/202. After crossing **Tariffville Rd./Rte. 315** (15.1 miles) at a trailhead, it parallels Rte. 10/202 and the **Farmington River** to **Simsbury** center where it joins a wooden guardrail separating **Iron Horse Blvd.** for a mile to **Drake Hill Rd.** (17.2 miles).

Here another detour ventures off the rail bed. Turning right on Drake Hill Rd., the trail heads uphill to Hopmeadow St./**Rte. 10/202**, turns left paralleling the roadway, then turns left into woods and descends back to the rail line. (Note that the intersecting **Stratton Brook Tr.** heads west from the opposite side of Hopmeadow St./Rte. 10/202.)

Continuing south, the trail straightens on the rail line for almost a mile, skirts a parking lot, and crosses Rte. 10/202 (19.0 miles) at **Sand Hill Rd.** It follows a utility line past a residential area and wetlands, intersecting **Latimer La.** (19.8 miles) and Rte. 10/202 (20.2 miles) along the way.

Approaching the center of **Avon**, the trail starts a 1.8-mile detour with a sharp right turn off the rail bed (21.3 miles) into woods. (Pavement also continues straight at this point to Mountain View Ave.) It soon crosses **Mountain View Ave.** and Rte. 10/202, parallels **Fisher Dr.** and **Ensign Dr.** on a separated pathway, then crosses Ensign on a marked, on-road route along **Climax Heights Rd.** At the end, a separated trail passes under **Rte. 44**, then another on-road route resumes turning right on **Darling Dr.** and left on **Security Dr.** Cross **Arch Rd.** and find the path on the left.

The rail-trail resumes with a faint uphill slope along a utility corridor and intersects **Country Club Rd.** (23.8 miles), **Scoville Rd.** (24.8 miles), and **Thompson Rd.** (25.3 miles). Entering Farmington, the slope then reverses as the trail descends across **Brickyard Rd.** (26.8 miles), crosses a bridge over **Rte. 4** (27.6 miles), and crosses the **Farmington River** on an especially long, high span (27.8 miles) shortly before the endpoint at **Red Oak Hill Rd.** (28.8 miles). Nearby to the west (right), the popular 10.2-mile **Farmington River Tr.** ventures upstream along the river.

BACKGROUND:

This route originated in 1836 as a canal between Northampton, MA and New Haven, CT. Over 80 miles in length, it was the longest ever built in New England and one of the most expensive requiring 28 locks to meet changes in elevation, 13 culverts to allow streams to flow underneath the canal, 3 aqueducts to carry the canal over rivers, and 135 bridges for roads. The canal struggled to generate revenue and closed in 1848 when a railroad was completed along the same route. After the railroad fell idle in the late 1980's, locals organized to create a recreational trail and construction of the first section started in 1994 in Connecticut. Additional trail construction is planned in both states and, utilizing the Manhan Rail-Tr. (Chapter 4), will eventually reconnect NorthamptonNew Haven.

DRIVING DIRECTIONS:

• **Shaker Farms Country Club trailhead, Westfield, MA:** From I-90 take Exit 3 and follow Rte. 10/202 south for 4 miles. Turn left on Tannery Rd. and drive for 0.5 miles, then turn left on Ponders Hollow Rd. (which becomes Shaker Rd.) and continue for 1 mile. After crossing the rail-trail, turn right at the country club and continue to the end of the road.

• **Rte. 20 trailhead, East Granby, CT:** From I-91 take Exit 40 and follow Rte. 20 west for 8.2 miles. Park in the lot at the Newgate Wildlife Management Area beside the trail.

• **Rte. 10/Rte. 315 trailhead, Simsbury, CT:** From I-91 take Exit 40 and follow Rte. 20 west for 9.4 miles to Granby. Turn left on Rte. 10 south and drive for 4.3 miles, then look for the trailhead on the left after the intersection of Rte. 315.

• **Brickyard Rd. trailhead, Farmington, CT:** From I-84 take Exit 39 and follow Rte. 4 west for 2.7 miles. Turn right on Brickyard Rd. and park in the lot 1 mile ahead on the left.

ADDITIONAL INFORMATION:

Friends of the Columbia Greenway, columbiagreenway.org
Friends of the Southwick Rail Trail, southwickrailtrail.org
Farmington Canal Rail-to-Trail Association, farmingtoncanal.org
Farmington Valley Trails Council, fchtrail.org

4 Manhan Rail-Trail, New Haven-Northampton Canal Line Trail

Southampton-Northampton

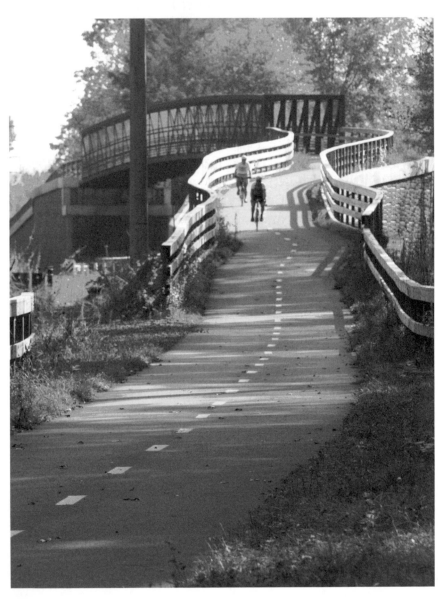

LENGTH: 9.6 miles
SURFACE: paved
TERRAIN: small slopes

Bridging roads and rivers, this three-pronged rail-trail is the southern spoke in Northampton's hub of options and will be part of a future interstate pathway to Connecticut.

RULES & SAFETY:
- Bicyclists should yield to pedestrians.
- Keep to the right, pass on the left, and alert others (*"On your left..."*) when approaching from behind.
- Dogs must be leashed and their wastes removed.
- Respect the private property along the trail.

ORIENTATION:

Millside Park in Easthampton serves as a central trailhead for the Manhan which extends in three directions from a nearby point. To the southwest, a 2.5-mile leg offers mostly shady conditions and passes through downtown Easthampton to neighboring Southampton. To the east, a 2.3-mile branch offers open surroundings near the Oxbow of the Connecticut River. To the north, a 4.8-mile ride enters Northampton where the trail is known as the New Haven-Northampton Canal Line and connects two other trails: the Francis P. Ryan Bikeway (Chap. 5) and the Mass. Central Rail-Tr./Norwottuck section (Chap. 6).

TRAIL DESCRIPTION:

Heading southwest on the Manhan from **Millside Park**, a 2.5-mile leg starts with a slight uphill slope past old mill buildings and an eastward view to Mt. Tom. It reaches downtown Easthampton at the crossings of **Union St.** (0.8 miles) and then **Payson Ave.** where the adjacent **Public Safety Complex** offers toilets and a water fountain. The trail returns to woods as it passes the Williston Northampton School, travels under **Park St.** (1.3 miles) at a high point, intersects **South St.** (1.8 miles), and currently ends just beyond the Southampton line at **Coleman Rd.** (2.5 miles).

Heading northeast from Millside Park, the Manhan

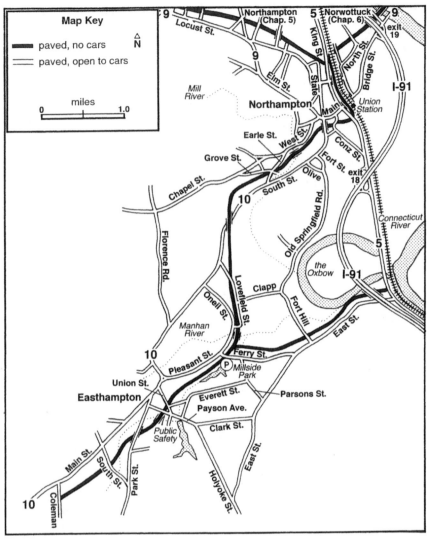

crosses **Ferry St.** and forks after a quarter-mile. The 2.3-mile eastern branch turns right from the main line just north of Ferry St., curving past an old mill building and descending on a slight downslope along a powerline to open surroundings near **Fort Hill Rd.** (1.0 mile). It parallels part of **the Oxbow**, once a sharp bend in the nearby **Connecticut River**, passes under **I-91** (2.0 miles), and ends at North St./**Rte. 5** (2.3 miles).

The trail's remaining leg continues northward over the

Manhan River, drops to **Lovefield St.** at a missing bridge (0.4 miles), then follows a utility line to a second crossing of Lovefield (1.1 miles). It enters Northampton as the **New Haven-Northampton Canal Line** and joins the edge of the former Farmington Canal for a short distance before rising on a long span across **Rte. 10** (1.9 miles).

Turning northeast, the trail traverses the intersection of **Earle St.** and **Grove St.** (2.7 miles), passes over the **Mill River** (3.2 miles), and turns left alongside Old South St. (3.7 miles) before crossing it. After intersecting **Pleasant St./Rte. 5** (4.0 miles), it curves north beside **Union Station**, parallels an active railroad, and crosses bridges over **Main St.** (4.2 miles) and **North St.** (4.5 miles). The trail ends (4.9 miles) at the junction of the **Francis P. Ryan Bikeway** (Chap. 5) which heads west (left) across Rte. 5 and the **Mass. Central Rail-Trail/Norwottuck section** (Chap. 6) which continues through a tunnel under the railroad.

BACKGROUND:

This route utilizes segments of two rail lines, the New Haven & Northampton which was completed in 1856 and the Easthampton Branch of the Connecticut River Railroad which was built in 1872. Both served the town's textile industry until the 1970's. Previously, the New Haven & Northampton line had been the route of the Farmington Canal, built in 1836 and measuring over 80 miles long.

When the trains stopped running, rail-trails were proposed and construction of the first section of the Manhan was completed in 2003. The trail has been extended southward to Southampton and northward to Northampton, and future construction will continue south to the Columbia Greenway in Westfield (Chap. 3).

DRIVING DIRECTIONS:

From I-91: Take Exit 18 and follow Rte. 5 south for 1.4 miles, turn right on East St. and drive for 1.5 miles, then turn right on Ferry St. and continue for 0.9 miles. Look for Millside Park on the left before the road ends at Pleasant St.

TOILETS:

Easthampton Public Safety Complex, Millside Park (seasonal)

ADDITIONAL INFORMATION:

Friends of the Manhan Rail Trail, manhanrailtrail.org
Friends of Northampton Trails and Greenways, fntg.net
Friends of Southampton Greenway, fofsg.org

5 Francis P. Ryan Bikeway

Northampton

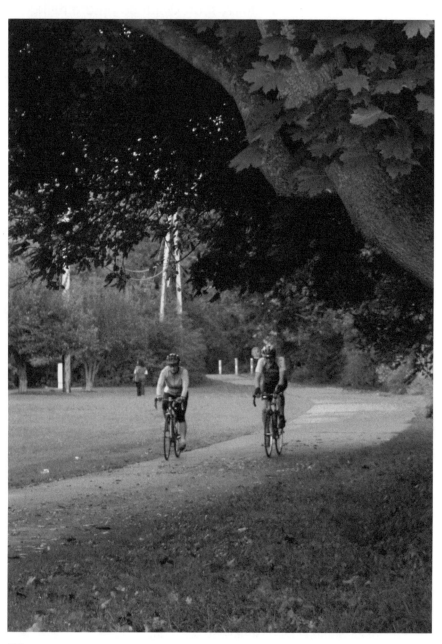

LENGTH: 5.6 miles
SURFACE: mostly paved
TERRAIN: gentle slopes
NOTE: parking fee required at Look Memorial Park trailhead

Decades of progress have created an admirable hub of rail-trails in Northampton. This bike path, the city's first, is a well-used link between the city center and outlying neighborhoods.

RULES & SAFETY:
- Bicyclists should yield to pedestrians.
- The posted speed limit is 10 m.p.h.
- Keep to the right, pass on the left, and alert others (*"On your left..."*) when approaching from behind.
- Use extra caution in the presence of children, pets, and horses since their movements can be unpredictable.
- Step off the trail when stopped so others can pass.
- Crosswalks and signs identify trail/road intersections. Stop before crossing and assume that drivers do not see you.
- Pets must be leashed and their wastes removed.

ORIENTATION:
The trail extends between the commercial area of King St/Rte. 5 in the southeast at the junction of the New Haven-Northampton Canal Line/Manhan Rail-Tr. (Chap. 4) the Mass. Central Rail-Tr./Norwottuck section (Chap. 6), and natural surroundings to the northwest. The lowest elevation is the southeast endpoint and the highest is the northwest.

Trailhead parking is available for a fee near the midpoint at Look Memorial Park, a private, 150-acre greenspace with toilets, water, and recreation facilities. Additional parking can be found on the adjoining Mass. Central Rail-Tr./Norwottuck section at Elwell State Park on Damon St. as described in Chap. 6.

TRAIL DESCRIPTION:
Heading southeast from **Look Memorial Park** toward downtown, 3 miles of trail begin by exiting the park at the main gate, crossing both **Rte. 9** and **Bridge Rd.** (0.2 miles) at

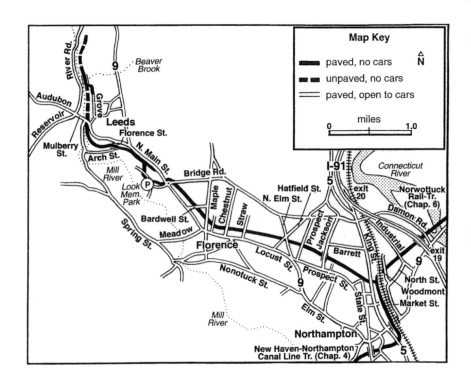

the rotary, and entering woods on the original railbed. The trail emerges at **Bardwell St.** (0.7 miles) at the village of **Florence** and curves eastward across a series of streets to **Straw Ave.** (1.3 miles), then returns to woods with a slight downward grade. It crosses the junction of **N. Elm St.** and **Hatfield St.** (1.8 miles), intersects **Prospect Ave.** (2.0 miles), then curves southeast under **Jackson St.** (2.3 miles) passing the Barrett St. Marsh on the left and connecting **State St.** on the right. The bikeway curves through a parking lot to a crosswalk at **King St./Rte. 5** (3.0 miles), turns north (left) alongside the busy roadway for a short distance, and then curves right to reach its terminus at the junction of two other rail-trails. To the right, the 9.6-mile **New Haven-Northampton Canal Line/Manhan Rail-Trail** (Chap. 4) extends toward downtown Northampton and Easthampton, and to the left the 10.9-mile **Mass. Central Rail-Tr./Norwottuck section** (Chap. 6) extends east through Hadley and Amherst.

Heading northwest from Look Memorial Park, the

bikeway extends for 2.6 miles. It begins paralleling the park's loop road past tennis courts and then crosses it, climbs to the rail bed (0.2 miles), and turns left beside **N. Main St./Rte. 9**. Just ahead it veers west alongside **Florence St.**, crosses a bridge over **Arch St.** (0.6 miles), and tilts upward on a noticeable incline as it curves north to a crosswalk at **Mulberry St.** (1.2 miles) in the village of **Leeds**.

The trail follows the **Mill River** upstream through woods with a variety of surfaces for the remaining 1.4 miles. A stone dust surface lasts until the intersection of a side trail (1.6 miles) ascending to **Grove Ave.**, then pavement resumes at a bridge over **Beaver Brook** (1.7 miles) and along a slope above the river. A dirt surface marks the final leg to the trail's endpoint (2.6 miles) at private property.

BACKGROUND:

Freight trains of the New York, New Haven, & Hartford Railroad used this route until 1969. A proposal to transform the corridor into a recreation trail was made a few years later and Northampton's bike path was open for use in 1984. Since that time, popularity for the trail spurred its expansion in both directions: east to Rte. 5 and the junction of the New Haven Northampton Canal Line/Manhan Rail-Tr. (Chap. 4) and northwest toward Williamsburg. The trail is named for a long-time Northampton DPW Director and City Engineer.

DRIVING DIRECTIONS:

Look Memorial Park from I-91 northbound: Take Exit 19, continue across Rte. 9 onto Damon St., drive for 1 mile to a Rte. 5 traffic signal, then continue straight on Bridge Rd. for 2.2 miles to a rotary at Rte. 9.   Enter the park on the opposite side, proceed downhill from the entrance booth, and park near the paved trail at the base of the slope.

Look Memorial Park from I-91 southbound: Take Exit 20 and merge onto Rte. 5 south. Turn right at the first traffic signal and follow Bridge Rd. for 2.2 miles to the end, cross Rte. 9 at the rotary to enter the park, then as above.

TOILETS:

Look Memorial Park, Elwell State Park (see Chap. 6)

ADDITIONAL INFORMATION:

Friends of Northampton Trails & Greenways, Inc., fntg.net
Look Memorial Park, lookpark.org, (413) 584-5457

6 Mass. Central Rail-Trail, Norwottuck section

Northampton-Belchertown

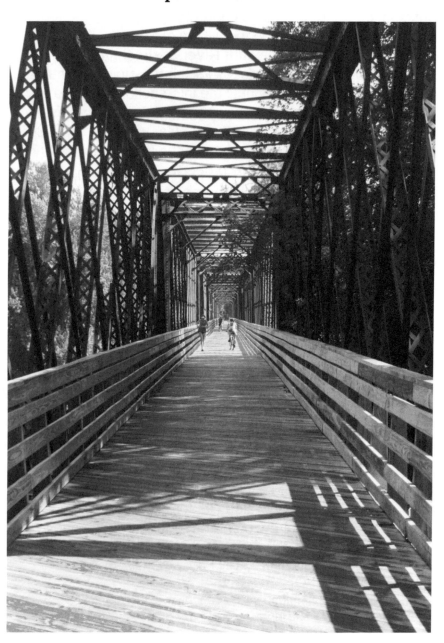

LENGTH: 10.9 miles, plus side trails
SURFACE: paved
TERRAIN: gentle slopes

Part of the Pioneer Valley's ever-expanding rail-trail network, this western leg of the Mass. Central unites the Amherst area with car-free commuting, recreation, and nature. A highlight is the trail's quarter-mile-long bridge across New England's biggest river.

RULES & SAFETY:
  • Bicyclists should yield to pedestrians.
  • Keep to the right, pass on the left, and alert others (*"On your left..."*) when approaching from behind.
  • Use extra caution in the presence of children and pets since their movements can be unpredictable.
  • Step off the trail when stopped so others can pass.
  • Respect nearby residents by keeping noise levels low.
  • Crosswalks and signs identify trail/road intersections. Stop before crossing and assume that drivers do not see you.
  • Pets must be leashed and their wastes removed.
  • Watch for additional information posted at trailheads.

ORIENTATION:
The trail has a mostly east-west alignment with numerous access points, including Elwell Recreation Area on Damon Rd. in Northampton which often fills to capacity.

Elevation changes are mild. The highest point is the midsection near Amherst center and low points exist near both ends. Mileage markers assist with plotting progress.

Adjoining trails include the UMass Bikeway which heads north from Amherst center and two trails which extend from the western endpoint in Northampton: the 9.6-mile New Haven-Northampton Canal Line/Manhan Rail-Trail heading south (Chap. 4) and the 5.6-mile Francis P. Ryan Bikeway (Chap. 5) heading northwest.

TRAIL DESCRIPTION:
Beginning at the **Elwell Recreation Area** trailhead, the Mass. Central/Norwottuck extends in two directions. To the

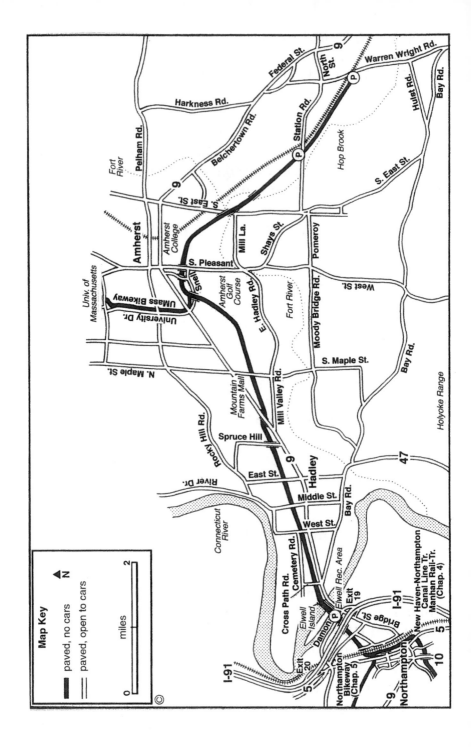

west, 0.8 miles of trail cross **Damon Rd.**, pass under **I-91**, intersect Bates St. and Woodmont Rd., and pass under an an active railroad. Turning left (south) on the other side, the trail parallels the tracks for a short distance before ending at the junction of the 9.6-mile **New Haven-Northampton Canal Line/Manhan Rail-Trail** (Chap. 4) straight ahead and the 5.6-mile **Francis P. Ryan Bikeway** (Chap. 5) on the right.

Heading east from Elwell Recreation Area, the Norwottuck extends for 10.1 miles through Hadley and Amherst to Belchertown. The ride begins with a view from a quarter-mile-long railroad trestle bridge spanning the **Connecticut River** and 60-acre **Elwell Island**. The trail traverses farmland on the other side and then a residential area where several roads intersect, including **West St.** at the long, slender common in **Hadley** center (1.8 miles). It passes underneath busy **Rte. 9** (3.1 miles) in a lighted tunnel where slopes and blind corners at both approaches require caution so ride at a safe speed and keep to the right side.

Resuming a straight line, the trail enjoys the shade of a tree canopy as it passes a mix of surroundings including farmland with distant views of the **Holyoke Range** as well as commercial areas with shopping centers and restaurants. Note that side trails branch to a few of these businesses including the **Mountain Farms Mall** (3.6 miles) where a designated trailhead parking area is provided and rest rooms are available.

The trail gains a faint uphill pitch after crossing **S. Maple St.** (3.9 miles) and the incline persists for the next couple of miles toward the center of Amherst. After crossing the Amherst town line it bends northward at the edge of the **Amherst Golf Course** which opens the scenery on the right. The **UMass Bikeway** intersects on the left after a bridge over **Snell St.** (5.5 miles) and extends north for almost 2 miles to the **University of Massachusetts** campus, first with a descent to a traffic signal at Rte. 9 and then in flat terrain and open surroundings beside **University Dr.**

Turning back to the east, the Norwottuck sinks below

ground level as it enters a cut at its highest elevation and passes under **S. Pleasant St./Rte. 116** (6.0 miles). Side trails climb to the roadway near **Amherst** center.

A slight downslope lasts for the next 2 miles as the trail turns southeast and straightens. It skirts tennis courts and playing fields of **Amherst College** on the left and then enters natural surroundings of farmland, wetland, and woods, much of it protected conservation land. More views of the Holyoke Range spread to the southwest along this stretch.

The trail crosses a pair of bridges over the **Fort River** and **S. East St.** (7.2 miles) where an unpaved side trail drops to a small trailhead on **Mill La.** After another bridge carries it over **Hop Brook** (7.6 miles), the trail proceeds through an expanse of wetland before reaching a larger trailhead parking lot at **Station Rd.** (8.6 miles).

The Norwottuck's last leg measures a mile and a half long and parallels a working railroad visible through trees on the left. Watch for a clearing in Lawrence Swamp which allows a final view of the Holyoke Range in the distance on the right. After crossing the Belchertown line, the trail reaches its eastern terminus at a trailhead parking lot on **Warren Wright Rd.** (10.1 miles).

BACKGROUND:

The Mass. Centrail Rail-Tr./Norwottuck section follows the route of the Massachusetts Central Railroad which began operating between Boston and Northampton in 1887. By the 1920's passenger service on the railroad had dwindled from increasing use of automobiles and ended in the 1930's during the Great Depression. Through service for freight continued until 1938 when a fierce hurricane washed out the tracks in Barre, but trains continued to use segments of the line until 1980.

Almost 100 years after its construction, the state purchased this western end of the line in 1985 in order to create a recreational trail and in 1992 construction was underway. The trail's Native American name means *"in the mist of the river"* and refers to the natives who inhabited the Connecticut River Valley.

Other segments of the original rail line are also used for recreation. Along the midsection the Mass. Central Rail-Trail is in use in Hardwick (Chap. 16), from Rutland to Barre (Chap. 17), and from Sterling to Holden (Chap. 18). At its eastern end the line is utilized by the Wayside Rail-Tr. in Wayland and Weston (Chap. 39) and the Fitchburg Cutoff Tr. in Cambridge and Belmont, the Red Line Linear Park in Cambridge, and the Community Path in Somerville (Chap. 40). Additional segments of the line have been either proposed or planned for conversion to trails.

DRIVING DIRECTIONS:

• **Elwell Recreation Area/Damon Rd. trailhead from I-91 northbound:** Take Exit 19 and continue straight at the end of the ramp (crossing Rte. 9) on Damon Rd. Look for the trailhead parking lot immediately ahead on the right.

• **Elwell Recreation Area/Damon Rd. trailhead from I-91 southbound:** Take Exit 20 and merge onto Rte. 5. Turn left at the first traffic signal on Damon Rd. and look for the trailhead parking lot on the left after one mile, just before the road ends at Rte. 9.

• **Warren Wright Rd. trailhead from I-90/Rte. 9 westbound:** Take Exit 8 and proceed to a traffic signal, turn right (on Thorndike St.) and drive for 0.7 miles, then continue west on Rte. 20 for 0.9 miles. Turn right on Rte. 181 and drive for 9.4 miles, continue north on Rte. 202 for 0.9 miles, then turn left on Rte. 9 west and drive for 5.6 miles. Turn left on North St. and continue for 0.6 miles, then turn left on Warren Wright Rd. and find the trailhead 0.6 miles ahead on the right.

• **Warren Wright Rd. trailhead from Rte. 9 eastbound:** Follow Rte. 9 east from the traffic circle near Amherst center for 4.3 miles. Turn right on North St. and continue for 0.6 miles, then turn left on Warren Wright Rd. and find the trailhead 0.6 miles ahead on the right.

TOILETS:

Damon Rd. trailhead, Mountain Farms Mall

ADDITIONAL INFORMATION:

Connecticut River Greenway State Park, (413) 586-8706
Dept. of Conservation & Recreation, mass.gov/dcr
masscentralrailtrail.org

7 Chicopee Memorial State Park
Chicopee

LENGTH: 2 miles
SURFACE: paved
TERRAIN: steep in places

Complementing a popular beach and picnic area, this short loop offers a hilly, curvy ride through nearby woods.

RULES & SAFETY:
- Bicyclists should yield to pedestrians.
- Compared to most bike paths, this route is relatively narrow, bumpy, steep, and curvy, so use appropriate caution.
- Ues extra caution near the beach and picnic area since it can be crowded.
- Dogs must be leashed and their wastes removed.
- An entrance fee is charged during summer.
- The posted closing time varies with the seasons so plan your stay accordingly.

ORIENTATION:
The paved trail starts at the parking lot, descends past the beach to a wooded area, and forks in a 1.5-mile loop. No other access point or intersections exist and few signs or markings are present along the trail.

TRAIL DESCRIPTION:
From the parking lot, descend the paved access road past the beach and along a row of shade trees on the southern shoreline of **Chicopee Reservoir**. After a third of a mile, the paved trail curves right and descends steeply to a bridge over **Cooley Brook**, then forks.

A 1.5-mile loop begins here. Turning left, the paved trail climbs for a quarter-mile then levels with a narrower width and a curvy course through woods. Near the midpoint, it turns eastward at the edge of **Westover Air Force Base** and parallels the boundary fence in a straight line, intersecting mountain biking paths which diverge into the

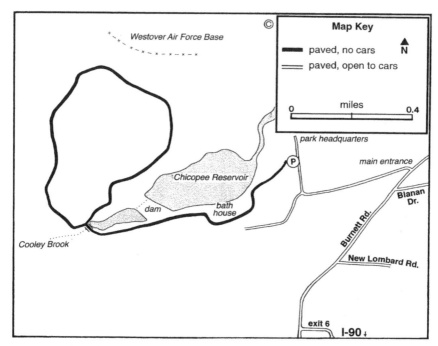

surrounding forest of pitch pines.

    Turning back to the south, the trail passes white birch trees as it emerges on a ridgeline above the reservoir, with the dam and beach visible through the woods. A final descent includes two especially steep pitches and several blind corners (use caution) and returns riders to the start of the loop. Turn left to return to the trailhead and beach.

BACKGROUND:

    Dedicated to the city's war veterans, Chicopee Memorial State Park preserves 574 acres for recreation at the outskirts of the city. Chicopee Reservoir, created in the early 1900's for water supply, is the park's centerpiece and serves as a popular swimming area in summer. The paved bike path was created in the early 1980's.

DRIVING DIRECTIONS:

    From I-90 (Mass. Tpke.): Take Exit 6. Leaving the toll plaza, turn right on Burnett Rd. (instead of left for I-291). The park entrance is a half-mile ahead on the left.

TOILETS:

trailhead

ADDITIONAL INFORMATION:

Chicopee Memorial State Park, (413) 594-9416

8   Connecticut River Bikeway
Springfield

LENGTH: 3.7 miles
SURFACE: paved
TERRAIN: flat

Springfield's riverfront includes a paved trail which is attractive to exercisers, railroad buffs, and basketball fans.

RULES & SAFETY:
- Bicyclists should yield to pedestrians.
- Keep to the right, pass on the left, and alert others (*"On our left..."*) when approaching from behind.
- Ride at a safe speed, especially at slopes and corners.
- Dogs must be leashed and their wastes removed.
- Note that the bike path has relatively few access points and is largely confined between the river and railroad.

ORIENTATION:
The Sullivan Visitor Information Ctr., just south of the Riverfront Park entrance, serves as a trailhead. Cross the railroad tracks and turn either north or south along the water.

TRAIL DESCRIPTION:
Turning south (left when facing the river) from the **Riverfront Park** entrance, cyclists can roll for 1.1 miles. The trail follows a narrow corridor lined by a tree-covered slope above the **Connecticut River** on one side and a chainlink fence bordering railroad tracks and **I-91** on the other. After a quarter-mile, a bike/pedestrian overpass bridges the tracks with access to the **Basketball Hall of Fame**. The trail ends before the **South End Bridge** with a view across the water to the confluence of the **Westfield River**.

Turning north (right when facing the river) from the park entrance, the riding lasts for 2.6 miles. It starts with a drop down a concrete ramp, slips under **Memorial Bridge**, then climbs a sloped bridge over railroad tracks and descends the other side in switchback turns. The trail joins a

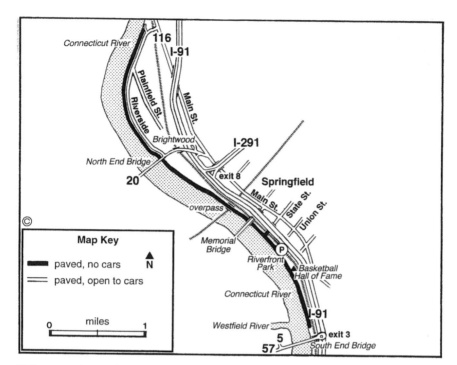

Map Key

▬▬ paved, no cars
══ paved, open to cars

▲ N

miles
0 ——————— 1

little-used roadway for a short distance, follows the top of a flood control dike, then intersects **Rte. 20** at the **North End Bridge** after 1.5 miles where a crosswalk and signal await.

The bikeway continues north into the residential area of **Brightwood** with a forested riverbank obscuring river views on the left and a concrete flood control dike rising on the right along **Riverside Rd.**, then ends at **Plainfield St.**

BACKGROUND:

The Connecticut River Bikeway opened in 2003. Its creation reclaimed river frontage that had been lost with the construction of the railroad, flood control dikes, and interstate highway and the trail enables easy access to nature from downtown Springfield. Future expansion has been proposed as part of a regional network of trails.

DRIVING DIRECTIONS:

• **I-91 northbound:** Take Exit 6, turn left on Union St., cross Hall of Fame Ave., and turn right at the visitor center.

• **I-91 southbound:** Take Exit 6, turn right at the next four-way intersection, and turn right at the visitor center.

Follow the sidewalk north from the parking lot to the intersection of State St., then turn left to enter the park.

9 Springfield Reservoir Trail
Ludlow

LENGTH: 3.2 miles (one way)
SURFACE: paved
TERRAIN: gentle slopes
NOTE: trail is closed on Wednesdays and certain holidays

Pristine lakeshore and forest surround this isolated, out-and-back trail with a uniquely peaceful setting. Its popularity can exceed its parking capacity on sunny days.

RULES & SAFETY:
• The area is managed for public water supply so strict rules are posted at the trailhead.
• Food is not allowed and littering is not tolerated.
• Dogs and other animals are not permitted.
• Skateboarding, in-line skating, and swimming are among the prohibited activities.
• Bicycliing is permitted only on the paved trail.
• Keep to the right, pass on the left, and alert others (*"On your left..."*) when approaching from behind.
• Be extra cautious in the presence of children since their movements can be unpredictable.
• A toilet is provided to protect the water supply.
• The area is closed on Wednesdays each week and on Thanksgiving, Christmas, and New Year's Day.
• The parking lot gate is locked each night. Closing time is posted at the trailhead and varies with day length.

ORIENTATION:
Accessible from only one endpoint, the trail intersects no roads and offers no other points of egress. It follows an isolated route along the reservoir's northern shoreline to a dead end, where trail users reverse direction and follow the same route back to the trailhead. Mileage markers are posted at points along the way but few other points of reference are evident.

TRAIL DESCRIPTION:

From the trailhead gate at the parking lot, the trail begins with a gentle downslope for a third of a mile to the first view of **Springfield Reservoir**. It continues past a toilet facility and **fishing pier** (0.5 miles) and curves through woods between the shoreline and the base of **High Hill**. Turning northward on a straight line, the trail enjoys more views over the water before reversing direction just past the 2-mile marker at the reservoir's northern reach. The remainder of the trail heads mostly south through more woods with fewer water views, then ends at a gated bridge (3.2 miles) beside a meadow on the reservoir's eastern shore.

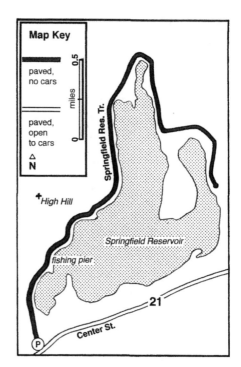

Reverse direction in order to return to the trailhead.

BACKGROUND:

Springfield Reservoir and the surrounding 1400-acre watershed are managed as a water supply area by Springfield's Water & Sewer Commission. The property opened to the public for limited passive recreation in 2002 following the state's purchase of a conservation restriction on the property which permanently preserves the land while also ensuring public access to it.

DRIVING DIRECTIONS:

From I-90 (Mass. Tpke.) take Exit 7 and follow Rte. 21 north for 3.4 miles. Look for the trailhead parking lot on the left just before the reservoir.

TOILETS:

beside the trail about a half-mile from the trailhead

ADDITIONAL INFORMATION:

Springfield Water & Sewer Commission, (413) 787-6256

10 Grand Trunk Tr., Trolley Tr.
Brimfield

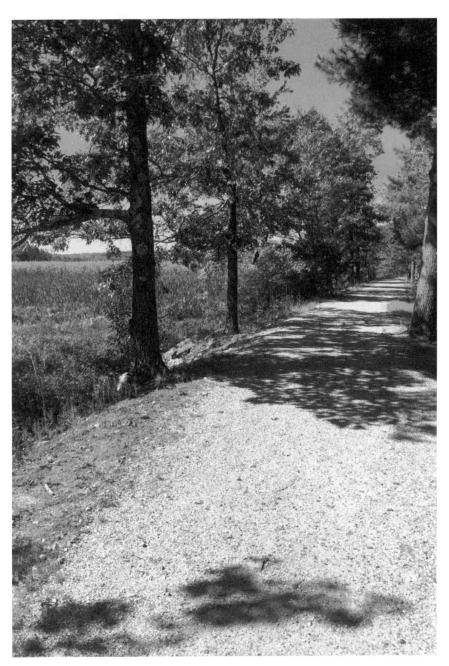

LENGTH: 5.3 miles (including side trails)
SURFACE: stone dust
TERRAIN: flat

Part of the so-called Titanic Rail-Trail, this old rail bed joins a parallel former trolley line and adjoining woods roads to provide a network of options for car-free biking in the natural surroundings of the Quinebaug River. Among the interesting sights is a vast forest scar left from a 2011 tornado.

RULES & SAFETY:
- Bicyclists should yield to pedestrians.
- Keep to the right, pass on the left, and alert others (*"On your left..."*) when approaching from behind.
- Be especially cautious in the presence of children and pets since their movements can be unpredictable.
- Pets must be leashed (6' max.) and wastes removed.
- Be careful not to block trailhead gates when parking.
- Visitors are asked to carry out all that they carry in.
- During periods of flooding the area can be closed.

ORIENTATION:

The Grand Trunk Tr. is actually a secondary route in this chapter and exists as fragments paralleling the main trail which was a former trolley line. Adjoining trails, also surfaced with stone dust, encounter modest slopes and include former roads closed as a result of the area's status as the East Brimfield Lake flood control area.

Most trails are well groomed with mowed borders, benches, interpretive signs, and other amenities. Sign posts provide a series of numbered points along the trails and are displayed on the map to assist visitors in determining their location. East Brimfield Lake's location points have the prefix EBL-GT along the Grand Trunk Tr. and the prefix EBL-LP along the Lake Siog Pass.

TRAIL DESCRIPTION:

Begin near the center of the trail network at the trailhead parking lot on **Five Bridges Rd.** Heading east (left when facing the rail bed), both the **Trolley Tr.** and the

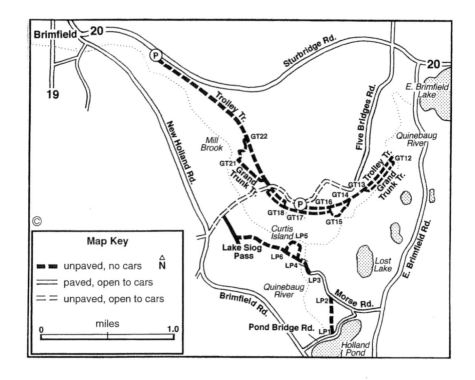

parallel **Grand Trunk Tr.** are visible crossing a nearby wetland. The Trolley Tr. (the left option) is the main route and extends for 0.9 miles to a missing bridge over the **Quinebaug River** while the Grand Trunk Tr. has a slightly rougher surface and is fragmented into several scenic loops along the river and its wetlands which offer worthwhile return-trip variations.

Heading west from the trailhead (right when facing the rail bed), the two trails split again before crossing Five Bridges Rd. The Trolley Tr. (the right option) curves northward through woods to reach a semi-open area damaged in a 2011 tornado, then straightens through an expanse of snapped tree trunks and regenerating forest to the **Rte. 20** trailhead (1.6 miles). Nearby, a half-mile loop veers away on another section of the Grand Trunk Tr. together with a new pathway that curves between trees.

The **Lake Siog Pass**, also known as the Holland Connector, starts on the other side of **Mill Brook** a half-mile south of the rail bed on Five Bridges Rd. The route begins at a gated road on the left, then forks left on a stone dust trail which crosses a wetland to **Curtis Island** and the Holland town line. Watch for an unsurfaced trail intersecting on the left which loops north with good views over surrounding wetlands. The main trail continues over a hill and follows the old pavement of **Morse Rd.** across a bridge over the Quinebaug River and uphill past another gate. Ride for another quarter-mile to a left-hand curve where a stone dust trail continues straight and descends to **Pond Bridge Rd.** and **Holland Pond** (also known as Lake Siog).

BACKGROUND:

The Grand Trunk Tr. follows the route of the never-completed Southern New England Railroad which was partially constructed between Palmer and Providence, RI from 1912 to 1915 by the Grand Trunk Railroad of Canada. Led by Charles Hays, who perished aboard the *Titanic* in 1912, the effort to build the ambitious, 85-mile route endured until World War I when financing became unavailable.

The parallel Trolley Tr. follows the route of an electric "interurban" trolley line which operated between Springfield and Worcester from 1907 until 1927 when automobile travel had gained popularity.

The surroundings are now managed as a flood control area centered on the E. Brimfield Dam. Following a severe flood in 1955, the U.S. Army Corps of Engineers established this and other dams to store excessive rainfall and prevent downstream catastrophes.

Developing these routes for recreation occurred over many years and was delayed by extensive destruction caused by a tornado in 2011. The Grand Trunk Tr. officially opened in 2013, and future development is expected to extend the rail-trail in both directions.

DRIVING DIRECTIONS:

From I-84 take Exit 3B and follow Rte. 20 west for 4.0 miles. Turn left on Five Bridges Rd. and continue for 1.6 miles to the trailhead parking lot on the left.

Alternatively, continue west on Rte. 20 for an additional 2 miles and find trailhead parking at a gate on the left.

ADDITIONAL INFORMATION:

U.S. Army Corps of Engineers, E. Brimfield Lake, (508) 347-3705

11 Grand Trunk Trail
Sturbridge-Southbridge

LENGTH: 2.1 miles, plus 0.8-mile side trail
SURFACE: stone dust
TERRAIN: small slopes

This section of the Grand Trunk rail bed visits Westville Lake's dam and flood control area, the Quinebaug River's rapids, and a large picnic area.

RULES & SAFETY:
- Bicyclists should yield to pedestrians.
- Keep to the right, pass on the left, and alert others (*"On your left..."*) when approaching from behind.
- Pets must be leashed (6' max.) and wastes removed.
- Visitors are requested to carry out all that they carry in.
- During periods of flooding the area can be closed.

ORIENTATION:
Located just uphill of the trailhead parking lot, the rail-trail heads west (left) with a flat, out-and-back option along the Quinebaug River and east (right) with a hillier loop option over the flood control dam and around Westville Lake. Sign posts along the trail have numbered location points (with the prefix WVL-GT) which are displayed on the map.

TRAIL DESCRIPTION:
Heading west (left) from the Sturbridge trailhead off **Breakneck Rd.**, the rail-trail follows a ledgy shelf on a slope above the **Quinebaug River** for the first 0.9 miles, with several bedrock cuts and pretty scenery of rocks and rapids. It then crosses the **Ed Calcutt Bridge** over the river and ends before reaching **River Rd.** (1.3 miles).

Heading northeast (right), the rail bed passes the **recreation area** and follows **Westville Lake** for 0.6 miles, then climbs and crosses the **dam** to the end of **Marjorie La.** (0.8 miles). Reversing direction, the 0.8-mile **Westville Lake Community Tr.** descends south into Southbridge on a hilly,

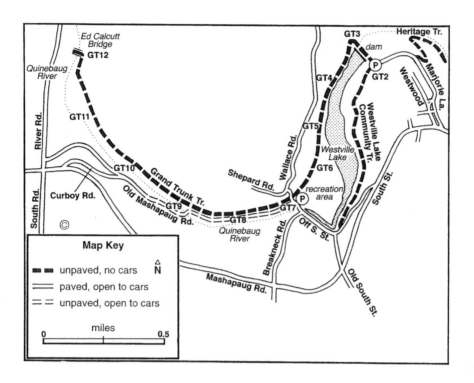

narrow course through woods with a stone dust surface ending at **Off South St.** Turn right to return to the trailhead (0.3 miles ahead) and complete a 1.9-mile loop.

BACKGROUND:

The Grand Trunk Trail follows the route of the never-completed S. New England Railroad which was partially constructed between Palmer and Providence, RI from 1912 to 1915. Sections of the line have been reborn as trails and this segment is envisioned to eventually link Rte. 15 in Sturbridge with West St. in Southbridge.

The U.S. Army Corps of Engineers built Westville Lake and Dam in 1962 in an effort to control the threat of flooding following severe damage from rains in 1955. During periods of flooding, the dam and its basin retain river water and later release it during safe periods.

DRIVING DIRECTIONS:

From I-84 take Exit 3B and follow Rte. 20 west. Turn immediately left on Rte. 131 east and continue for 2.3 miles, then turn right on Wallace Rd. Drive for 0.9 miles, turn left at the Westville Lake sign, and park in the first lot on the left.

ADDITIONAL INFORMATION:

U.S. Army Corps of Engineers, E. Brimfield Lake: (508) 347-3705

12 Quinebaug River Rail-Trail
Dudley-Southbridge

LENGTH: 5.4 miles, in two parts
SURFACE: gravel, crushed stone, grass
TERRAIN: flat
NOTE: mountain bikes advised

Rough in places, this rural rail bed lies in two parts offering river scenery, natural surroundings, and solitude.

RULES & SAFETY:
- Road intersections have no crosswalks.
- Pets must be leashed and their wastes removed.
- Hunting occurs near the trail so wear blaze orange clothing in late fall. In Dudley, the trail is closed to dogs during deer shotgun season (late November to mid-December). Hunting is prohibited by state law on Sundays.

ORIENTATION:

The 4.2-mile western leg in Dudley and Southbridge has appealing scenery along the Quinebaug River for much of the way while the 1.2-mile eastern leg in Dudley is less remote. If unmarked side trails create confusion, rely on the rail bed's flat, steady course for guidance.

TRAIL DESCRIPTION:

The 4.2-mile western leg is accessed from **Mill Rd.** in Dudley. Heading northwest, it enters a gravel pit after a mile where several other trails intersect, then straightens through woods to a closed bridge at the **Quinebaug River** (1.9 miles) where bicyclists detour to the right on a side path and turn left on **W. Dudley Rd.** in order to cross the water. Resuming on the right at an old factory beside **W. Dudley Pond**, the trail continues upstream into Southbridge as the surface degrades from grass to gravel and then to large-size crushed stone, slowing the last 0.9 miles of riding to **Rte. 131** (3.9 miles).

The 1.2-mile eastern leg is accessed from **Schofield**

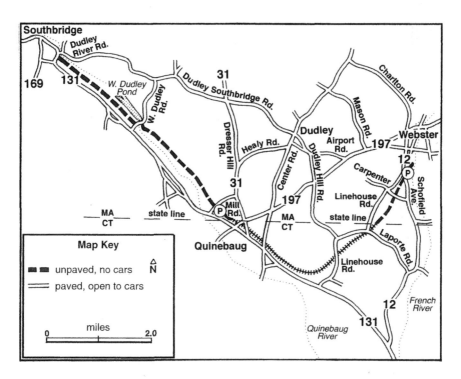

Ave./Rte. 12 in Dudley. Work continues on the midsection but the northern end offers a view of the **French River** and the southern end visits the Boston Rd. Conservation Area.

BACKGROUND:

Built in 1859, this route originated as the Boston, Hartford, & Erie Railroad and operated until 1982. The state acquired it for use as a recreational trail in 2004 and town personel have led the process of removing rails and ties, rebuilding bridges, and installing amenities. Future work is hoped to unite and extend the existing trail segments.

DRIVING DIRECTIONS:

Mill Rd.: From I-395 take Exit 2 and follow Rte. 16 west to the first traffic signal. Continue straight on Rte. 12 south for 1.6 miles, then continue straight on Rte. 197 south for 3.5 miles (into CT). Turn right on Rte. 131 and drive north for 0.5 miles (back to MA), then turn right on Mill Rd. Look for the trailhead a short distance ahead on the right.

Schofield Rd.: From I-395 take Exit 2, follow Rte. 16 west to the first traffic signal, then Rte. 12 south for 2.5 miles. Look for the trailhead parking lot on the left.

13 Quabbin Reservation
Petersham, Hardwick

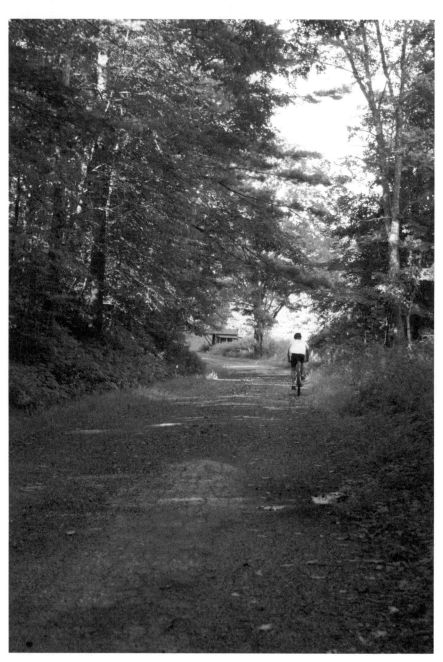

LENGTH: 10.3 miles
SURFACE: varies between old pavement and gravel
TERRAIN: hilly
NOTE: wide-tired bicycles recommended

Loaded with the solitude of a 55,000-acre wilderness, these old roads explore the long-abandoned town of Dana.

RULES & SAFETY:
• Bicycling is permitted only on designated roads and is prohibited elsewhere (watch for signs).
• The area is managed for water supply so strict rules apply: no swimming, wading, walking on ice, etc.
• Dogs and horses are restricted from the reservation.
• Do not block trailhead gates when parking since work crews and emergency vehicles always need access.
• Portable toilets are provided at numerous locations. Disposing of human wastes anywhere else is prohibited.
• Watch for additional rules posted at trailheads.

ORIENTATION:
Few signs of civilization are present so pay careful attention to the map when exploring for the first time. Many of the road names are posted together with intersection numbers which are displayed on the map to assist visitors with determining location.

TRAIL DESCRIPTIONS:
Starting from **Gate 40** at **Rte. 32A**, **Dana Rd.** leads up a small hill and then levels between stone walls, relics of former farmland now shaded by forest. After passing an arm of **Pottapaug Pond**, visible through trees on the left, the road reaches the site of **Dana Common** (1.8 miles) where a former village was abandoned in 1938 to ensure a clean watershed for the reservoir. Today old shade trees, the town common, and foundations are the only remains.

Three roads reach beyond this clearing but their surface conditions degrade with sections of either gravel or grass. Branching left at intersection **40-5**, little-used **Thayer Rd.** runs south for a mile through woods to a peninsula on

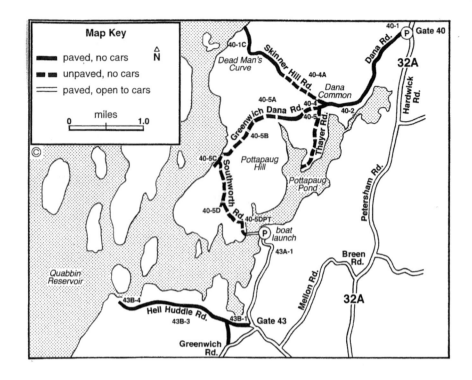

Pottapaug Pond. The first half is mostly gradual uphill and the second half is mostly downhill.

Forking right from Dana Common, 1.6-mile **Skinner Hill Rd.** is a more strenuous option heading northwest to another shoreline view. It begins with a slight downslope to a stream and then tilts upward on a mile-long climb between stone walls and old maples. The road finally crests and descends a 0.6-mile drop to the reservoir with a sharp, right turn known as **Dead Man's Curve** deserving caution halfway down. The old asphalt surface remains intact for most of this downhill before it disappears beneath the water.

Continuing straight (west) from Dana Common, 2-mile **Greenwich Dana Rd.** links additional routes for biking. After passing an arm of Pottapaug Pond, it follows stone walls through more woods with a mix of ups and downs and surfaces alternating between old pavement and gravel. It parallels the reservoir for a short distance before ending at another shoreline view.

Southworth Rd. forks left at intersection **40-5C** just before this endpoint. Its gravel surface climbs for the first third of a mile, traverses a slope of **Pottapaug Hill**, and forks left at **40-5D** before descending back to the reservoir at a **boat launch** and rental area after 1.5 miles.

Continue across the dam and ride the access road (open to cars) south for 1.7 miles to **Gate 43** where **Hell Huddle Rd.** runs west with another 2.1 miles of car-free pedaling. It holds smooth pavement and sizeable slopes before ending abruptly at a chainlink fence, 9.1 miles from the Gate 40 trailhead on Rte. 32A.

BACKGROUND:

Named with the Nipmuc word for *land of many waters*, Quabbin Reservoir was constructed between 1926 and 1939 and flooded 39 square miles with an average of 50' of water. Four towns were abandoned from the reservoir area and its surrounding watershed including Dana, settled in 1735, which had been a prosperous community of farms, small industries, and summer estates. Dana's general store, town hall, school, church, 15-room hotel, and many residences were either torn down or moved.

Quabbin Reservoir supplies water to nearly half the state's population throughout the metropolitan Boston area by a series of aquaducts and pipelines spanning the 60-mile distance. Careful management involves engineers testing the water, foresters and biologists monitoring the woodlands, and officers patrolling the area.

DRIVING DIRECTIONS:

Gate 40 from I-90: Take Exit 8 and follow Rte. 32 north. After 13 miles bear left on Rte. 32A and continue north for 8.5 miles to the trailhead on the left.

Gate 40 from Rte. 2: Take Exit 17 and follow Rte. 32 south for 6 miles. Turn right (west) on Rte. 122 and drive for a half-mile, then turn left (south) on Rte. 32A and continue for 3 miles to the trailhead on the right.

TOILET FACILITIES:

Portable toilets are provided at numerous locations including: Gate 40, Dana Common, boat launch area.

ADDITIONAL INFORMATION:

Quabbin Visitors Center, (413) 323-7221
Friends of Quabbin, foquabbin.org

14 Ware River Trail
Barre-Templeton

LENGTH: 13.0 miles
SURFACE: gravel, rough in places
TERRAIN: flat
NOTE: wide-tired bikes advised

This old railroad grade is now a gated, and somewhat bumpy, dirt road venturing through the shade and solitude of remote woods.

RULES & SAFETY:
• Use caution when crossing roads since crosswalks are not present. Assume that drivers do not see you.
• Be self-sufficient in food, water, and bike repair tools since the trail reaches remote areas.
• Note that parts of the trail traverse a water supply area where special rules for usage are posted.
• Hunting is permitted along much of the trail so wear blaze orange clothing during deer season in Nov. and Dec.
• Be careful not to block trailhead gates when parking.

ORIENTATION:
The Rte. 122 trailhead (southern terminus) is the trail's lowest elevation and recommended starting point. Natural scenery dominates the entire trail but is best between Williamsville Rd. and Stone Bridge Rd. where ponds and wetlands open otherwise forested surroundings.

TRAIL DESCRIPTION:
Beginning at **Rte. 122** in Barre, the rail-trail heads north from a metal gate into a vast woodland paralleling the **Ware River**. After 1.8 miles it crosses a gravel road which descends to the confluence of the **Burnshirt River**, then continues along an ungated segment that parallels **Grainger Rd.** to **Rte. 62** (2.9 miles). Use caution when crossing Rte. 62 since it has fast traffic, limited visibility, and no crosswalk.

The trail parallels **Gilbert Rd.** for the next 1.2 miles

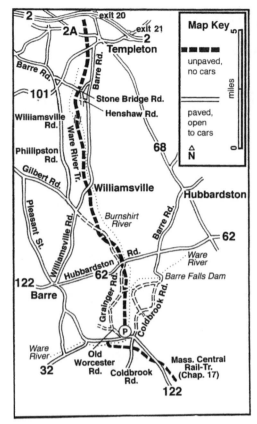

and enjoys deep woods until **Williamsville Rd.** (6.0 miles), which also deserves caution when crossing. The next 4.1-miles include views of Williamsville Pond (6.5 miles) and an open wetland at a bridge over the Burnshirt River (8.8 miles).

North of **Stone Bridge Rd.** (10.1-miles) the surface conditions degrade. The trail crosses **Rte. 101** (11.6 miles) near the center of **Templeton**, intersects **Rte. 2A** (12.1 miles) at a former industrial site, and dead-ends near **Rte. 2** (13.0 miles).

BACKGROUND:

The Ware River Railroad began operation in the 1870's between Palmer and Winchendon. Both passenger and freight service ended by the 1960's, the rails and ties were removed soon after, and the state later acquired the route for use as a recreational trail.

DRIVING DIRECTIONS:

From I-90: Take Exit 8 and follow Rte. 32 north for 21.3 miles to S. Barre, turn right on Vernon Ave. and continue for 1 mile, then turn right (south) on Rte. 122. Drive for 1.4 miles to the trailhead on the left before a bridge at the Oakham town line. Find the rail-trail up the slope.

From Rte. 2: Take Exit 21 and follow Rte. 101 south for 1.5 miles. After Templeton center, turn left on Barre Rd. (which becomes Williamsville Rd. in Barre) and continue fo9.7 miles to Barre center. Turn left (south) on Rte. 122 and drive for 4.5 miles to the trailhead on the left before a bridge.

15 North Central Pathway
Winchendon-Gardner

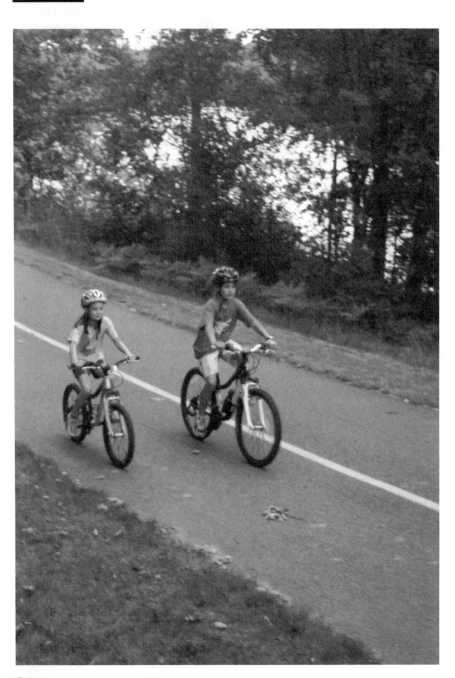

LENGTH: 9.4 miles in three parts, plus on-road connections
SURFACE: mostly paved, some gravel, some rough dirt
TERRAIN: gentle slopes

Mostly rail-trail, this three-part bike path holds pristine scenery and relatively few road intersections but requires on-road riding between each of the three sections.

RULES & SAFETY:
- Bicyclists should yield to pedestrians.
- Keep to the right, pass on the left, and alert others (*"On your left..."*) when approaching from behind.
- Be especially cautious in the presence of children and pets since their movements can be unpredictable.
- Stop at road intersections and remember that drivers might not be aware of your presence.
- Pets must be leashed and their wastes removed.

ORIENTATION:
The North Central Pathway exists in three separate sections, each with its own trailhead. The 2.9-mile northern section is a rail-trail with excellent water views along the Millers River. The 3.3-mile midsection is also a rail-trail with deep woods scenery and adjoins rougher paths along undeveloped sections of the rail bed at both ends for additional riding with wide-tired bikes. The 0.8-mile southern section is not a rail-trail and rolls and turns beside a lake.

TRAIL DESCRIPTION:
Beginning on the northern section at **Glenallan St.** in Winchendon, the pathway heads in two directions. To the north, it briefly leaves the rail bed to curve with the shore of **Whitney Pond**, crosses a bridge above a dam at the pond's outlet, and ends at playing fields off **Summer St.** near downtown (0.8 miles). To the south, the trail begins with a slight uphill slope to the edge of **Rte. 12**, parallels the edge of the roadway for a quarter-mile, then veers away from the traffic on a straight line to **N. Ashburnham Rd.** (2.1 miles). Open wetlands and three bridges over the **Millers River** allow pretty views along the way.

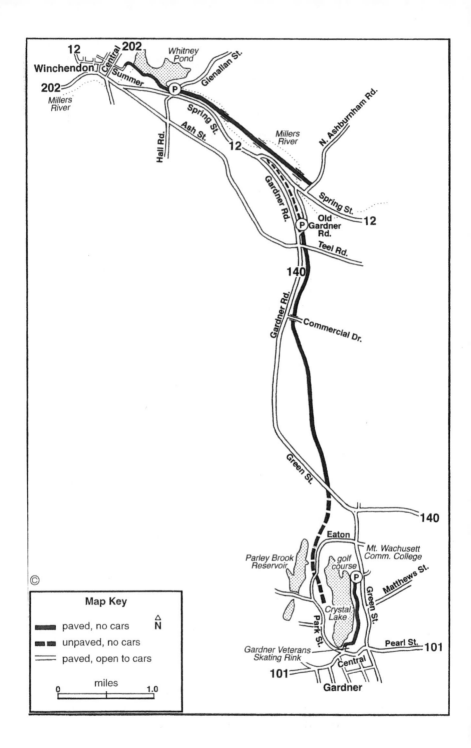

A 1.8-mile on-road route links the next section of trail. Turn right on N. Ashburnham Rd., right on Spring St./Rte. 12, and immediately left on **Old Gardner Rd.**, then ride for 1.5 miles to the trail crossing. Turning right (north), 0.8 miles of undeveloped rail-trail connect Rte. 12 with narrow, rough surfaces that require a mountain bike. Turning left (south), 3.3 miles of paved trail explore a vast area of woods, crossing **Teel Rd.** (0.2 miles), rising on a gradual, mile-long slope with a tunnel under **Commercial Dr.** (1.0 mile), then flattening in deep woods. After entering Gardner (2.1 miles), The paved trail crosses an open wetland and tilts slightly downhill to **Green St./Rte. 140** (3.3 miles) where it ends.

The rail bed continues south with an undeveloped, gravel surface for another 1.6 miles but requires caution when crossing the Rte. 140's high speed traffic. The trail passes a power substation (3.7 miles), climbs gradually across **Park St.** (4.5 miles), and then dead-ends (4.9 miles).

Nearby, the **Crystal Lake** trailhead serves a woodsy, 0.8-mile section of pathway linking the **Gardner Veterans Skating Rink** with short slopes and pretty water views.

BACKGROUND:

The North Central Pathway utilizes several different routes. The northern segment originated as the Cheshire Railroad in 1847 between S. Ashburnham and Bellows Falls, VT. The middle segment originated as the Boston, Barre, & Gardner Railroad and was built in 1874. Rail use ceased by the 1960's, rail-trail proponents organized in 1995, and trail construction has progressed in phases since 1997. Future trail construction is expected to extend from Gardner to the New Hampshire border where other trails already exist.

DRIVING DIRECTIONS:

• **Glenallan St. trailhead:** From Rte. 2 take Exit 24B and follow Rte. 140 north for 9.7 miles, then continue straight on Rte. 12 north for 1.5 miles and park in the lot on the right.

• **Old Gardner Rd. trailhead:** From Rte. 2 take Exit 24B and follow Rte. 140 north for 8.7 miles. Turn right on Old Gardner Rd. and immediately left at the parking lot.

• **Crystal Lake trailhead:** From Rte. 2 take Exit 24B and follow Rte. 140 north for 4.6 miles. Turn left on Green St. and find the trailhead 1 mile ahead on the right.

16 Mass. Central Rail-Trail
Hardwick-New Braintree

LENGTH: 2.7 miles
SURFACE: stone dust, mowed grass
TERRAIN: flat

This short segment of the Mass. Central explores rural farm fields and quiet woods along the Ware River.

RULES & SAFETY:
- Bicyclists should yield to pedestrians.
- Keep to the right, pass on the left, and alert others (*"On your left..."*) when approaching from behind.
- Pets must be under control at all times and pet wastes must be removed.
- Swimming is prohibited.
- Hunting is permitted so take appropriate precautions in November and December, the most popular period.
- Motorized vehicles are prohibited, but snowmobiles are allowed in winter.
- The trail is open from sunrise to sunset.

ORIENTATION:
The trail extends in two directions from the Depot Rd. trailhead to endpoints at paved roads, and has no other access points. Natural scenery is equally good along the entire length.

TRAIL DESCRIPTION:
Heading northeast (across **Hardwick Rd.**), the trail's straight line has a smooth, stone dust surface which is needle-covered from surrounding pines. It crosses a bridge over the **Ware River** (0.4 miles) and ends after another half-mile at the intersection of **Pine St.** and **Maple St.** (0.9 miles).

Heading southwest (across **West Rd.**), the stone dust follows a wooded corridor past a few fields, crosses a bridge over the Ware River (0.7 miles), then reverts to mowed grass. After crossing a smaller bridge over a farm road, the

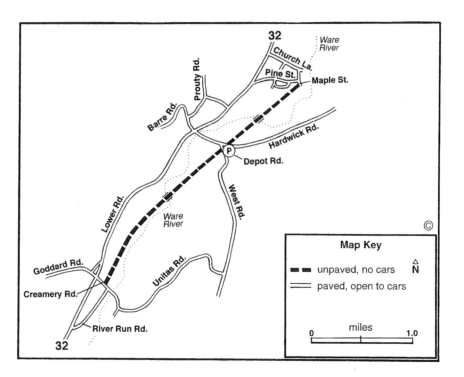

trail bends left paralleling an active railway, which is barely visible through trees, and ends at **Creamery Rd.** (1.8 miles).

BACKGROUND:

The Massachusetts Central Railroad was completed in 1887 along a 100-mile route between Boston and Northampton. The line thrived during its early years but suffered damage at its midsection from the Hurricane of 1938 and was never repaired. By the 1980's almost the entire line was inactive.

The East Quabbin Land Trust originated in 1994 to protect the area's farmland, wildlife habitat, and other resources. The group purchased 3.2 miles of the rail bed in 2007 and opened this section as a recreational trail in 2015. Additional work is planned.

DRIVING DIRECTIONS:

From I-90, take Exit 8 and follow Rte. 32 north for 17 miles to a four-way intersection. Turn right on Hardwick Rd. and cross the Ware River, fork right on West Rd., then immediately left on Depot Rd. and park by the trail sign.

ADDITIONAL INFORMATION:

East Quabbin Land Trust, eqlt.org
masscentralrailtrail.org

17 Mass. Central Rail-Trail
Rutland-Barre

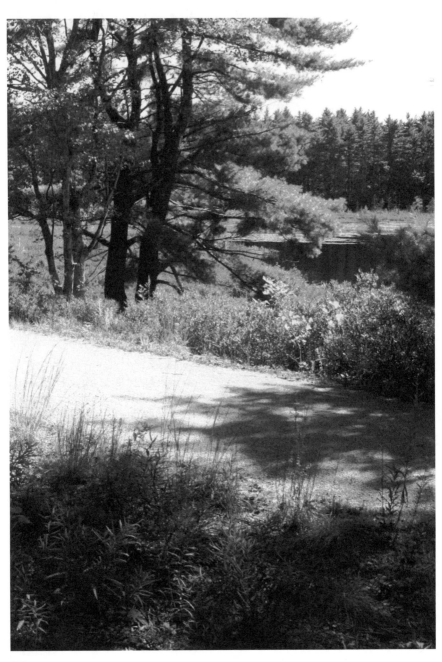

LENGTH: 8.5 contiguous miles, plus (additional) nearby
SURFACE: stone dust
TERRAIN: small slopes, except for the western endpoint

Spine of the state's future rail-trail network, the expanding Mass. Central is a work-in-progress worth visiting. This section combines miles of natural surroundings with a smooth, stone dust surface.

RULES & SAFETY:

- Bicyclists should yield to pedestrians.
- Keep to the right, pass on the left, and alert others (*"On your left..."*) when approaching from behind.
- Much of the trail is located in a public water supply area. Any act that pollutes the water supply is prohibited.
- Dogs are excluded from many areas. Where dogs are allowed, their wastes should be removed.
- Hunting is permitted in some areas so wear blaze orange clothing during deer season in Nov. and Dec.

ORIENTATION:

The trail has an east-west alignment with many trailheads providing access. Elevation change is minimal with the lowest point at the western end. Natural scenery is best along the midsection where numerous ponds and wetlands open otherwise forested surroundings.

TRAIL DESCRIPTION:

Beginning at the **Miles Rd.** trailhead in Rutland, the trail runs in two directions. Heading east, a 1.6-mile leg curves up a slope from the parking area past the Wachusett Greenways **Welcome Center** and headquarters. The trail continues across the road and soon joins the route of the Massachusetts Central Railroad, passing under **Rte. 56** and following the edge of **Moulton Pond** and several wetlands on the way to **Glenwood Rd.** (1.6 miles).

An additional 1.4-mile trail segment begins southeast of nearby **Wachusett St.** To reach it, turn right on Glenwood and ride uphill for 0.7 miles, then turn left on Wachusett and find the trail after 1.3 miles on the right, just before **Rte. 68.**

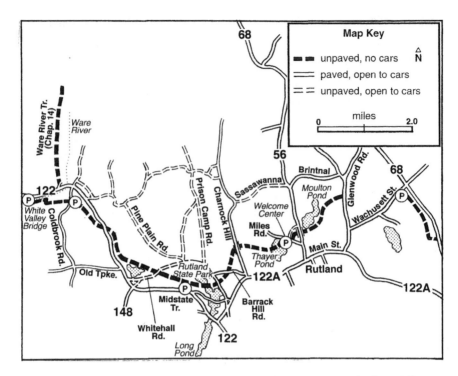

Map Key

■ ■ unpaved, no cars

─── paved, open to cars

═ ═ unpaved, open to cars

Heading west from the Miles Rd. trailhead, the riding stretches for 6.9 miles. The trail begins on a causeway through **Thayer Pond** and surrounding wetland, then enters woods and rises on a slight slope through a long bedrock cut to an underpass at **Charnock Hill Rd.** (1 mile). Leveling, it intersects gravel-surfaced **Barrack Hill Rd.** (1.6 miles) and a slight downslope develops as the trail enters **Rutland State Park**, a popular summer destination for swimming.

The trail takes a minor detour at a missing bridge over **Whitehall Rd.** (1.9 miles), dropping on a moderate slope to cross the street and returning uphill to the rail bed. It then reaches one of its most scenic parts, a high causeway built between **Long Pond** and Whitehall Pond which are visible through trees on both sides. Continuing into woods, it passes the **Midstate Trail** parking area on the left.

After a second crossing of Whitehall Rd. (3.2 miles), the trail enjoys more water and wetland views at Muddy Pond where it enters Oakham and turns north near the side of **Rte. 122**. Trees shield the trail from the nearby roadway.

The trail intersects Rte. 122 (4.8 miles) at a sign warning of high speed car traffic, so use caution when crossing. Separating from the roadway on the other side, it enjoys quiet forest scenery to **Coldbrook Rd.** (5.6 miles), site of a former rail depot and now a trailhead parking lot.

The final leg turns westward for another half-mile before diverting from the Mass. Central rail bed near the Barre town line, descending a slope with switchback turns, and joining the grade of the former Ware River Railroad along the **Ware River** for a short distance. Heading downstream, the trail passes a spillway at a water supply building, descends from the rail bed to a bridge over the river, and ends at Rte. 122 (6.9 miles) a short distance from the southern end of the **Ware River Tr.** (Chap. 14).

BACKGROUND:

Completed in 1887, the Massachusetts Central Railroad ran for 100 miles from Boston to Northampton. The line thrived during its early years but its midsection was destroyed by a hurricane in 1938 and was never rebuilt. By the 1980's most of the line was inactive.

Wachusett Greenways, a volunteer group, originated in 1995 with the vision of connecting this region with trails and greenways and has been the driving force behind the creation of the Mass. Central Rail-Tr. The group has raised awareness for the project, organized construction efforts, and helps maintain the trail. Future improvements are planned and contributions are welcome.

DRIVING DIRECTIONS:

Miles Rd. trailhead from I-190: Take Exit 3 and follow W. Mountain St. toward Holden. After about 1 mile turn left at a traffic signal on Shrewsbury St. and drive for 0.8 miles, then turn right on Rte. 122A North and continue for 7.2 miles to Rutland center. Turn right on Rte. 56 North and drive for 0.3 miles, then bear left on Miles Rd. Trailhead parking is 0.3 miles ahead on the left side of the road.

TOILETS:

Miles Rd. at the Wachusett Greenways Welcome Center (just up the hill from the trailhead), Midstate Trailhead at Rutland State Park

ADDITIONAL INFORMATION:

Wachusett Greenways, www.wachusettgreenways.org
masscentralrailtrail.org

18 | Mass. Central Rail-Trail
W. Boylston, Holden, Sterling

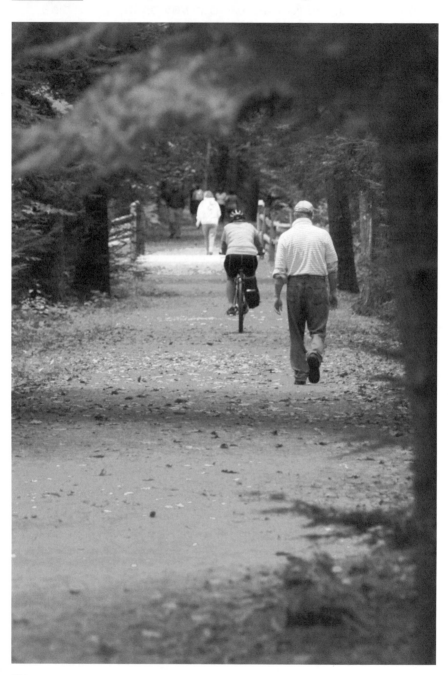

LENGTH: 7.4 miles, plus 2 miles of on-road connections
SURFACE: stone dust, gravel
TERRAIN: gentle slopes on rail bed, plus a few hilly detours
NOTE: mountain bikes advised on hilly detours

This section of the Mass. Central holds a variety of conditions along a combination of rail bed sections, detours on forest roads, and on-road links. Soothing forest scenery along the Quinapoxet River is especially beautiful.

RULES & SAFETY:

- Bicyclists should yield to pedestrians.
- Keep to the right, pass on the left, and alert others (*"On your left..."*) when approaching from behind.
- Much of the trail is located in a public water supply area so any act that pollutes the water supply is prohibited.
- Dogs are excluded from many areas so watch for signs. Where dogs are allowed, wastes should be removed.
- Hunting is permitted in some areas so wear blaze orange clothing during deer season in Nov. and Dec. Hunting is prohibited by state law on Sundays.

ORIENTATION:

This chapter involves two separate sections of rail-trail which have easy biking on smooth, stone dust surfaces. On-road routes and adjoining forest roads link the rail-trails although sloped terrain and rougher surfaces make the forest roads more difficult to ride. The W. Boylston trailhead offers a central location and direct access to a 2.8-mile section of rail-trail and the Sterling trailhead provides access to a 1.6-mile section. Trailheads have alpha-numeric identifications (shown on the map) with prefixes WB marking West Boylston locations, H for Holden, and S for Sterling.

TRAIL DESCRIPTION:

Beginning at the **Thomas St.** trailhead (**WB30**) in W. Boylston, 2.8 miles of smooth stone dust head west along the rail bed with excellent scenery along the riffles and rapids of the **Quinapoxet River**. The trail crosses under **I-190** (1.3 miles) at the Holden town line then passes stone ruins of the

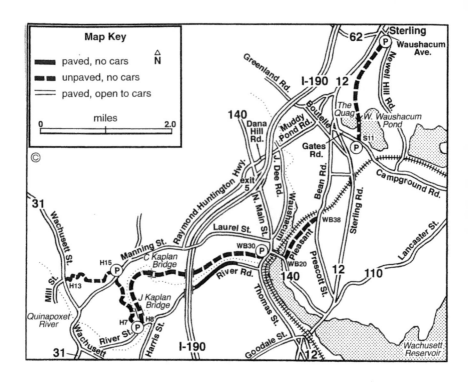

Springdale Mill (1.6 miles) on the left. It enjoys views of the river from the **Charlotte Kaplan Bridge** (1.8 miles) and the **Jeremiah Kaplan Bridge** (2.7 miles) before ending at **H8** and a trailhead parking lot on **River St.** (2.8 miles).

Here a more challenging 2.1-mile trail continues off the rail bed with hilly terrain and a stone dust surface which has minor erosion on several slopes. Starting from **H7** at the trailhead parking lot, this forest road climbs a few short pitches, descends to a field and crosses **Manning St.** (3.7 miles) at another trailhead parking lot (**H15**), then tackles a bigger uphill with switchback turns. It flattens at the top along a utility corridor before dropping abruptly to **H13** at **Rte. 31** (4.9 miles from the Thomas St. trailhead).

Heading east from the Thomas St. trailhead in W. Boylston, bicyclists follow a 3-mile on- and off-road route to reach another section of rail-trail. Turn left on Thomas St., right on **Rte. 140** (0.1 miles), cross the **Wachusett Reservoir**, then turn left at **WB20** (0.3 miles) on a gated gravel road known as **Pleasant St.** which continues into woods beside stone walls. Climbing over a hill, this old road lasts for almost a mile to **WB38** at **Prescott St.** (1.2 miles) where another on-road route links the next segment of rail-trail. Turn left on Prescott St. (which becomes **Bean Rd.** in Sterling) and ride for 1.2 miles, turn right just before Rte. 12 on **Gates Rd.** (2.6 miles) and ride for 0.3 miles (crossing Rte. 12 along the way). Look for the rail-trail on the left at **S11** across from a small trailhead parking lot (2.9 miles).

Heading north, this 1.6-mile branch line off the Mass. Central has a smooth, stone dust surface, keeps to flat terrain, and enjoys an excellent water view from a bridge between **the Quag** and **W. Waushacum Pond.** It ends at a trailhead parking area at a former railroad depot off **Waushacum Ave.** near **Sterling** center.

BACKGROUND:

The Massachusetts Central Railroad, completed in 1887, ran a 100 miles from Boston to Northampton. The line thrived in its early years but its midsection suffered destruction from the Hurricane of 1938 and was never rebuilt. By the 1980's most of the line was idle.

Wachusett Greenways, a volunteer group, originated in 1995 with the vision of connecting the region with trails and has been the driving force behind this rail-trail's development, raising money and awareness for the project, managing trail construction efforts, and making future plans for improvements.

DRIVING DIRECTIONS:

W. Boylston trailhead from I-190: Take Exit 5 and follow Rte. 140 south for 1 mile. Where Rte. 140 turns left at an intersection, keep straight on Thomas St. and then turn immediately right at the trailhead parking lot.

Sterling trailhead from I-190: Take Exit 6 and follow Rte. 12 south for 1.8 miles to Sterling center. Turn left on Waushacum Ave., cross School St., and look for the trailhead on the right, beyond the old depot building.

TOILETS:

W. Boylston and Sterling trailheads, in season

ADDITIONAL INFORMATION:

Wachusett Greenways, www.wachusettgreenways.org
masscentralrailtrail.org

19 Depot Trail
Spencer

LENGTH: 1.7 miles
SURFACE: stone dust
TERRAIN: noticeable slopes

Nestled in rolling countryside west of Worcester, this not-so-flat rail-trail is free of road intersections as it explores truly quiet surroundings of woods and wetlands.

RULES & SAFETY:
- Bicyclists should yield to pedestrians.
- Keep to the right, pass on the left, and alert others (*"On your left..."*) when approaching from behind.
- Pets must be leashed and their wastes removed.
- Be careful not to block the trailhead gate when parking since emergency vehicles always need access.
- Respect the private property along the trail.
- Motorized vehicles are prohibited, except for snowmobiles in winter.
- The trail is open from dawn until dusk.

ORIENTATION:
Parking for the Depot Trail is available at the southwest end on S. Spencer Rd. The trail encounters no road intersections and access is limited to the two endpoints. Natural scenery dominates the entire length with the highlight being open wetland along the Cranberry River.

TRAIL DESCRIPTION:
Heading northeast from the **S. Spencer Rd.** trailhead, the **Depot Trail** immediately tilts downward on a slight slope shaded by pine forest. Near the bottom it intersects a rough trail on the right venturing south into bordering **Spencer State Forest**, then flattens beside an open floodplain at the **Cranberry River** (0.4 miles).

Rising back into pine forest on the other side, the trail begins a gentle incline which lasts for the remaining 1.3

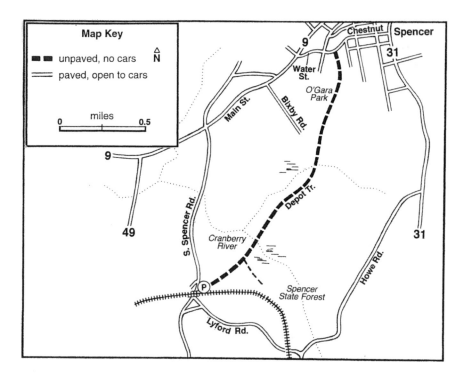

miles. It crosses a second stream and smaller wetland as it curves northward, passes under a powerline (1.3 miles) near the **O'Gara Park** baseball field, and then comes within sight of a few homes before ending at **Chestnut St.** (1.7 miles) near the center of **Spencer**.

BACKGROUND:

This route originnated in 1879 as the Spencer Branch of the Boston & Albany Railroad, a 2-mile branch line linking the center of Spencer to the main line at S. Spencer. It provided passenger service until the Great Depression and freight service until 1972, when the line was abandoned. Three decades later, a local effort secured grants from the state's Recreational Trails Program and performed clearing, drainage work, and surfacing for the trail.

DRIVING DIRECTIONS:

From I-90, take Exit 9 and follow I-84 south to exit 3A. Drive east on Rte. 20 for 2.0 miles, then turn left on Rte. 49 and continue north for 3.8 miles. Turn right on Flagg Rd., which becomes S. Spencer Rd., and watch for the small trailhead parking lot 3 miles ahead, just after an underpass.

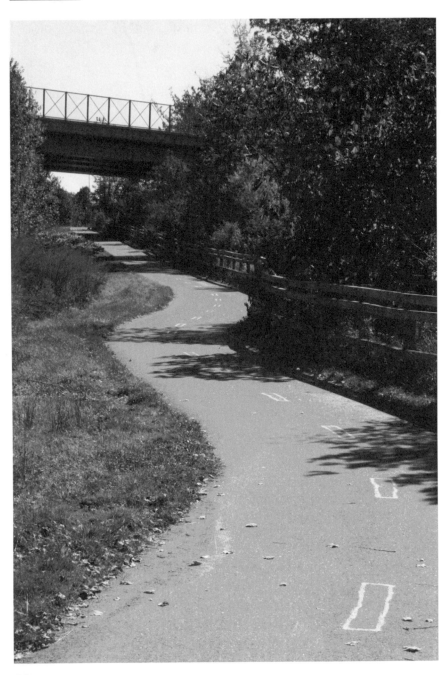

LENGTH: 2.9 miles
SURFACE: paved
TERRAIN: small hills

Bound for Providence, this first leg of a future regional trail threads intricately between streets, two highways, a railroad, and river. Amazingly, it intersects only two roads.

RULES & SAFETY:
  • Bicyclists should yield to pedestrians.
  • Keep to the right, pass on the left, and alert others (*"On your left..."*) when approaching from behind.
  • Be especially cautious in the presence of children and pets since their movements can be unpredictable.
  • The bike path encounters hills, curves, bumps, and overgrowing foliage so ride at a safe speed.
  • Stop at road intersections and remember that drivers might not be aware of your presence.
  • Pets must be leashed and their wastes removed.

ORIENTATION:
The trail's short length and lack of road intersections make it difficult to get lost although its complex route over and under numerous bridges can be disorienting. Side trails branch to nearby roads at several points.

Construction is underway on another half-mile of trail at the northern end and will include a new visitor center off McKeon Rd. which will serve as an excellent point of access.

TRAIL DESCRIPTION:
Starting at the **Millbury St.** trailhead in Worcester, the bike path heads north (right when facing the trail from the parking lot) for 1.4 miles toward the city. It follows the **Blackstone River** underneath **Rte. 146**, continues beside railroad tracks for a half-mile, then dips under a bridge for **Blackstone River Rd.** (0.7 miles) at a side trail to **Tobias Boland Way**. The trail continues past a shopping center before ending at **McKeon Rd.** (1.4 miles) where construction of a visitor center and another half-mile of trail to the campus of Holy Cross is underway.

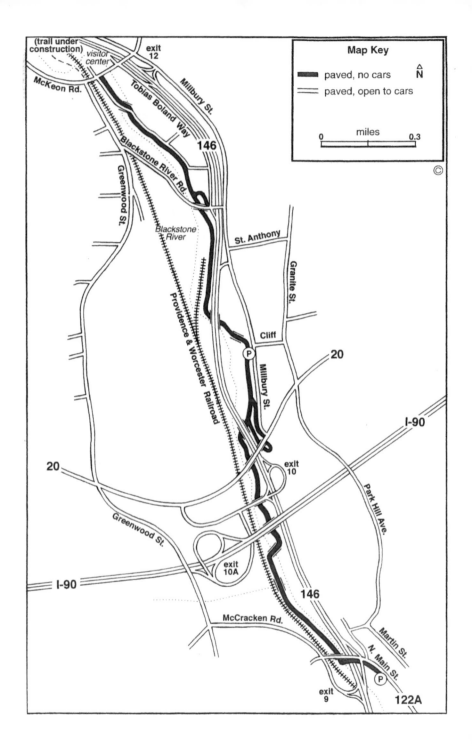

Map Key

━━━ paved, no cars
═══ paved, open to cars

Ṋ
N

0   miles   0.3

(trail under construction)
visitor center
exit 12
McKeon Rd.
Millbury St.
Tobias Boland Way
146
Blackstone River Rd.
Greenwood St.
Blackstone River
Providence & Worcester Railroad
St. Anthony
Granite St.
Cliff
P
Millbury St.
20
20
I-90
Park Hill Ave.
exit 10
Greenwood St.
exit 10A
I-90
146
McCracken Rd.
Martin St.
N. Main St.
P
exit 9
122A

©

Heading south (left when facing the trail from the Millbury St. parking lot), the bike path runs for 1.5 miles toward Millbury. The ride begins with an uphill beside Millbury St. and forks right at the top where a spur continues straight to connect the westbound side of **Rte. 20**. The trail descends past a trail serving Rte. 20 eastbound, then joins the edge of the river and passes under Rte. 146. Entering Millbury, it rises and falls with small slopes over the next half-mile and winds under 3 more bridges, joining the riverbank at several points. After passing under **I-90** (0.7 miles) and over the Blackstone, the trail enjoys a leafy corridor paralleling the **Providence & Worcester Railroad** and crosses a bridge over a side channel (1 mile) along the way. It passes under **Main St.** (1.3 miles), rises on a large bridge spanning the river and **Rte. 146**, intersects an **Exit 9** off-ramp at a crosswalk and signal, and descends to the southern terminus and trailhead parking lot at **Rte. 122A** (1.5 miles).

BACKGROUND:

The Blackstone River played an important role in America's early industrial history, providing power for mills (including the first to spin cotton in 1790) as well as the water for a canal linking Worcester and Providence in 1822. To honor this heritage, Congress established the Blackstone River Valley National Corridor in 1986 with the plan for a 50-mile greenway to extend from Worcester to Providence, RI. Most of this section was created in 2005 in conjunction with a highway construction project. Other sections include 3.7 miles in Uxbridge, Millville, and Blackstone (Chapter 21) and 10 miles in Rhode Island from Woonsocket to Cumberland.

DRIVING DIRECTIONS:

• **Millbury St., Worcester trailhead from I-290:** Take Exit 12 and follow Rte. 146 south. Take Exit 12, turn left off the ramp on McKeon Rd., then right on Millbury St. Look for the trailhead parking area 1.4 miles ahead on the right.

• **Rte. 122A, Millbury trailhead from I-90:** Take Exit 10A and follow Rte. 146 south. Take exit 9 for Rte. 122A south, turn right at the end of the ramp, and look for the trailhead parking lot 0.2 miles ahead on the right.

ADDITIONAL INFORMATION:

Blackstone River Valley Nat'l Heritage Corridor, www.nps.gov/blac

21 Blackstone Valley Greenway
Blackstone-Uxbridge

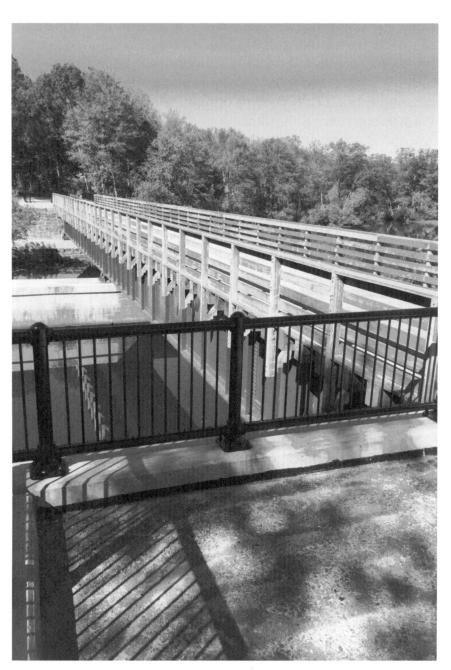

LENGTH: 3.8 miles
SURFACE: paved
TERRAIN: flat

This new section of the Blackstone doubles as the middle leg of the Southern New England Trunkline Tr. and will be the junction of a future 3-state bike path network. Four bridges along the route allow river views.

RULES & SAFETY:
- Bicyclists should yield to pedestrians.
- Keep to the right, pass on the left, and alert others (*"On your left..."*) when approaching from behind.
- Pets must be leashed and their wastes removed.
- The trail is open from sunrise to sunset.

ORIENTATION:
The trail's eastern half has river views from bridges in Blackstone and Millville while the western half has mostly wooded surroundings in Millville and Uxbridge. The lowest elevation is the Canal St. trailhead in Blackstone and the highest is the Millville Lock trailhead in Millville. Unmarked, on-road routes are required to link 3 other rail-trails nearby.

TRAIL DESCRIPTION:
Starting at the eastern end at **Canal St.** in Blackstone, the trail extends in two directions. Heading east (left when facing the trail from the parking lot), it runs for only 0.1 miles over a **St. Paul St.** bridge near the Rhode Island **state line**.

Heading west (right when facing the trail), it extends for 3.7 miles through Blackstone, Millville, and Uxbridge. Bridges dominate the first 1.5 miles starting with a high span over the **Blackstone River** and continuing with a cluster of shorter ones over roads including **Main St./Rte. 122** (0.2 miles). After passing under Church St., the trail emerges on a bridge over a section of the river which once served as the Blackstone Canal (0.5 miles). It continues across a third bridge over the river (0.7 miles) and makes a straight line to an underpass at Main St./Rte. 122 (1.3 miles) before entering Millville. Just ahead, it reaches the so-called **Triad**

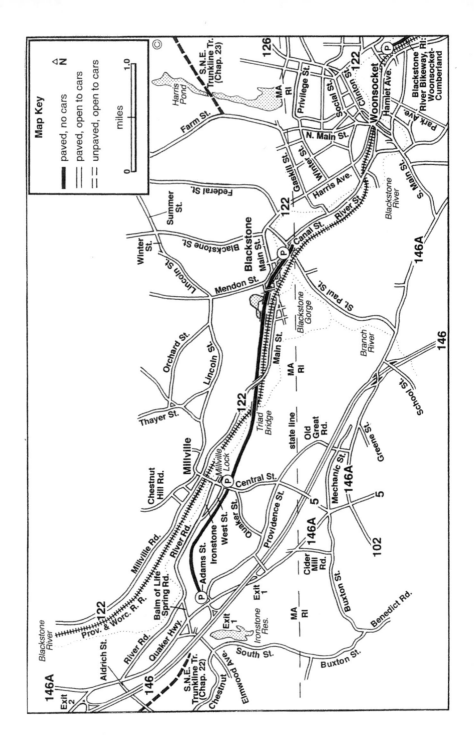

Bridge (1.5 miles) where 3 railroads cross the river at 3 different heights: the still-active **Providence & Worcester Railroad** occupies the lowest bridge, the rail-trail utilizes the middle level, and the never-completed Grand Trunk Railway's abutments and piers rise to the highest elevation.

Rising on a slight incline through woods, the trail reaches its highest point at the **Millville Lock** trailhead (2.4 miles) at **Central St.** before tilting downward on the other side. After crossing the Uxbridge town line, it passes under a powerline (3.3 miles) and diverts off the rail bed near **Rte. 146A** to a trailhead on **Adams Dr.** (3.7 miles).

BACKGROUND:

Birthplace of the Industrial Revolution, the Blackstone River was hailed *the hardest working river* for its use as a power source and transportation route. This history is honored by a 45-mile national heritage corridor extending from Worcester to Providence including a recreational greenway planned for most of the way. Other completed sections include a 2.9-mile segment in Worcester and Millbury (Chap. 20) and a 10-mile segment in Rhode Island from Woonsocket to Cumberland. Originating in 1854 as the Boston & New York Central Railroad, this section of the greenway also serves as part of the Southern New England Trunkline Tr. (see chapters 22 and 23).

DRIVING DIRECTIONS:

Blackstone trailhead from I-495: Take Exit 18 and follow Rte. 126 south for 8 miles. After crossing the state line at Woonsocket, RI, turn right on Rte. 114 north (Privilege St., which becomes Winter St.) and drive for 1.4 miles to the end. Turn right on Rte. 122 north and drive for 0.8 miles to enter Blackstone, MA, then turn left on St. Paul St., right on Canal St., and left at the entrance to the trailhead parking lot.

Uxbridge trailhead from Rte. 146 southbound: Take Exit 1, turn right on Rte. 146A, turn right on Providence St., and left on Adams St. Park in the lot ahead on the right.

Uxbridge trailhead from Rte. 146 northbound: Take Exit 1, turn right on Rte. 146A, turn left on Providence St., and left on Adams St. Park in the lot ahead on the right.

ADDITIONAL INFORMATION:

Blackstone Heritage Corridor, blackstoneheritagecorridor.org
Friends of the SNETT, facebook.com/snettfriends/

S. New England Trunkline Tr.
Airline State Park Tr.
Uxbridge-Thompson, CT

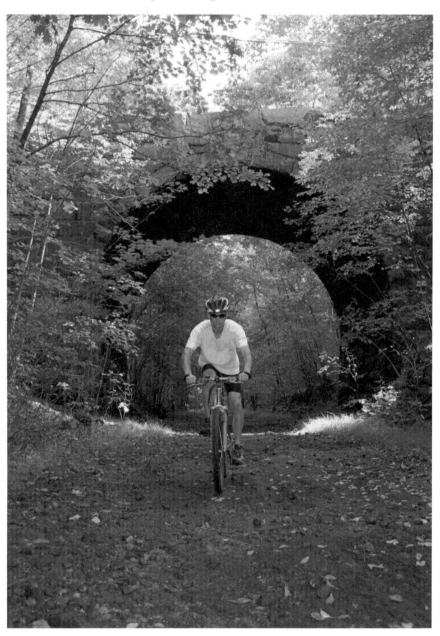

LENGTH: 18.1 miles
SURFACE: gravel, crushed stone
TERRAIN: slight slopes, steeper at some road intersections
NOTE: wide-tired bikes advised

      The revitalized SNETT and Connecticut's Airline Tr. combine for an especially long ride. Pristine scenery along the midsection includes a swimming beach in summer.

RULES & SAFETY:
- Bicyclists should yield to pedestrians.
- Keep to the right, pass on the left, and alert others (*"On your left..."*) when approaching from behind.
- Crosswalks are not present. Stop at all roads and remember that drivers might not be aware of your presence.
- Use extra caution where missing bridges create steep slopes at some road intersections.
- Respect nearby residents by keeping noise levels low.
- Pets should be leashed and their wastes removed.
- When encountering horses, bicyclists should use extra caution. Stop at the side of the trail and make verbal contact with the rider so that the animal will feel safe.
- Hunting is permitted along the trail so wear blaze orange clothing from mid-October through December. Note that hunting is prohibited by state law on Sundays.
- Motorized vehicles are prohibited.
- Watch for additional information posted at trailheads.

ORIENTATION:
      The trail offers woodsy surroundings along its entire length with the midsection at Douglas State Forest being the scenic highlight as well as the longest section without road intersections. The state forest is also home to a swimming beach in summer, toilets, and trailhead parking.
      The trail's lowest elevations are the endpoints near the Quinebaug River in the west and the Blackstone River in the east, and the highest elevation is the midpoint at Wallum Lake Rd.'s stone arch bridge in Douglas State Forest. Remember that starting from the trailhead near this high

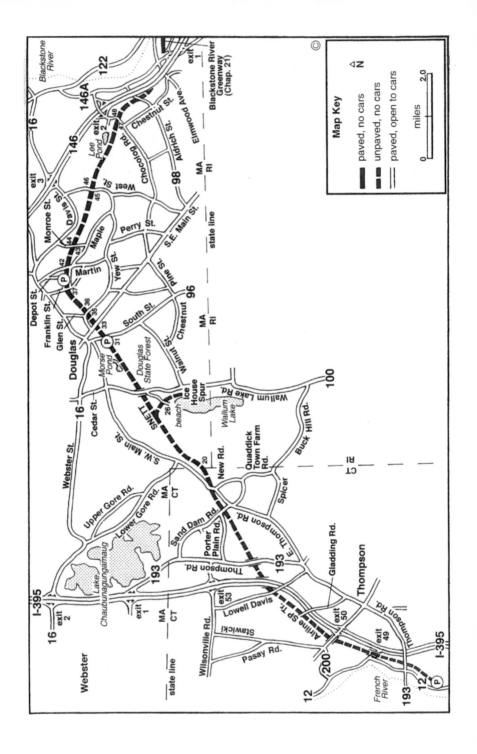

point requires a more difficult, uphill return ride.

The trail surface varies and is destined to improve along some sections. Wide-tired bikes are advised because much of the trail has a coarse surface of gravel and a few sections have loose or bumpy conditions. At several locations, the route's original bridges are now missing so the trail negotiates abrupt slopes in order to cross roads. Trailhead gates at road intersections along the midsection of the trail are numbered and displayed on the map to assist visitors in tracking their location.

Nearby rail-trails utilize other sections of this rail line. To the east, the Blackstone River Greenway (Chapter 21) continues from a point beyond Rte. 146 in Uxbridge to Blackstone and the SNETT (Chapter 23) is open from Blackstone to Franklin. To the west, the Airline State Park Tr. in Connecticut resumes beyond Thompson with 53 miles of riding south of Putnam.

TRAIL DESCRIPTION:

Heading southwest from the **South St./Rte. 96** trailhead (at gate 31, away from the road) in Douglas, the **Southern New England Trunkline Tr. (SNETT)** extends across 5,000-acre **Douglas State Forest** as the first leg of an 11.3-mile route into Connecticut. A faint uphill slope brings the trail past **Morse Pond**, between bridge abutments for the never-finished Grand Trunk Railway, and under a stone arch bridge carrying **Wallum Lake Rd.** (1.5 miles) at the trail's high point.

Here it leaves the Blackstone River watershed and enters the Quinebaug with a slight downhill slope for the remaining distance. Wetlands and ponds open the scenery along the next few miles as the trail straightens across the state forest, intersecting footpaths and mountain biking trails along the way. Watch on the left for the **Ice House Spur** (2.3 miles), a bumpier, 0.8-mile rail-trail to the shore of **Wallum Lake** intersecting the state forest's **beach** access road at gate 26.

Leaving the open wetlands along Rocky Brook, the

SNETT descends to gate 20 (3.9 miles) where it crosses the Connecticut state line and becomes the **Airline State Park Tr.** Just ahead, watch for a footpath on the left which extends for 0.3 miles to the Tri-State Marker at the junction of Massachusetts, Rhode Island, and Connecticut.

The Airline State Park Tr. descends abruptly at the crossing of **E. Thompson Rd.** (4.5 miles) where a bridge has been removed, then climbs a banking to cross **Sand Dam Rd.** (5.2 miles) where a bridge site has been filled. Flattening for the next mile and a half, the trail struggles with a loose, crushed stone surface in several areas before passing under **Thompson Rd./Rte. 193** (6.7 miles) and **I-395** (7.3 miles). It curves southward and parallels the highway with traffic noise becoming noticeable at **Lowell Davis Rd.** (7.5 miles) and persisting for the next few miles.

The trail intersects **Gladding Rd.** (8.3 miles), passes under **Rte. 200** (9.1 miles), and detours left off the rail bed at a missing bridge over a stream just before it crosses a bridge over the on/off-ramps for **exit 49** (10.0 miles). Processed stone covers the remaining distance as the trail dips to intersect **Thompson Rd./Rte. 193** (10.6 miles), parallels the **French River**, and ends at a trailhead parking lot beside Riverside Dr./**Rte. 12** (11.3 miles).

Heading northeast from the **South St./Rte. 96** trailhead (at gate 32, across the road), the SNETT extends for 7.5 miles with a few rough spots and a slight downslope. The trail intersects 6 roads in the first 2.7 miles as it skirts the center of **Douglas** and turns southeast, passing another trailhead at **Depot St.** (1.8 miles) along the way. After crossing **Monroe St.** (2.7 miles) at gates 43 & 44, the trail contends with areas of berms and a coarse, crushed stone surface as it enters Uxbridge, and drops on an eroded slope to **West St.** (4.1 miles) at gates 45 & 46.

Smooth riding resumes on the other side and the trail traverses deep woods until **Lee Pond** (5.2 miles) opens a view on the left. Crossing **Chockalog Rd.** (5.9 miles) at gates 47 & 48, it narrows and encounters areas of poor drainage and rough surface on the way to **Aldrich St./Rte. 98** (6.7 miles), then dead-ends beside the 4 lanes of **Rte. 146** (7.5 miles).

The **Blackstone Valley Greenway** (Chap. 21) begins 2 miles away. To reach it, follow Aldrich St./Rte. 98 downhill (east) for 0.4 miles (passing under Rte. 146), turn right on Rte. 146A and continue for 1.4 miles, turn left on Providence St. for 0.1 miles, then turn left on Adams St. and look for the trailhead on the right.

BACKGROUND:

The Boston & New York Central Railroad began operating along this route from Boston to Thompson, CT in 1854. The line extended to New York in 1874 on a direct, "air line" from Boston with express trains making the trip in record times. A 1955 flood destroyed the railroad's bridge over the Quinebaug River in Putnam, CT and a 1968 flood destroyed a bridge over the Blackstone River in Blackstone, ending through service.

Massachusetts and Connecticut later acquired portions of the route for recreation, and trail improvements have been progressing in stages. Other rail-trails utilizing this rail line include the Blackstone Valley Greenway from Uxbridge-Blackstone (Chap. 21), the S. New England Trunkline Tr. from Franklin-Blackstone (Chap. 23), and the Airline State Park Tr. in Connecticut from Putnam to East Hampton.

DRIVING DIRECTIONS:

• **Rte. 96, Douglas from I-495:** Take Exit 19 if northbound or 20 if southbound and follow Rte. 16 west for 17 miles to Douglas. Turn left on Rte. 96 south and continue for a half-mile to the trailhead parking on the right.

• **Rte. 96, Douglas from I-395:** Take Exit 2 and follow Rte. 16 east for 6.8 miles, turn right on Rte. 96 south, and continue for a half-mile to the trailhead on the right.

• **Rte. 12, Thompson, CT from I-395:** Take Exit 50 and follow Rte. 200 west for 1 mile to the end. Turn left and follow Rte. 12 south for 2.3 miles and watch for the trailhead on the left.

TOILETS:

Douglas State Forest boat ramp

ADDITIONAL INFORMATION:

Douglas State Forest, (508) 476-7872
Friends of SNETT, facebook.com/snettfriends/

23 S. New England Trunkline Tr.
Franklin-Blackstone

LENGTH: 5.3 miles
SURFACE: mostly gravel, varies from smooth to rough
TERRAIN: flat, with slopes at several road intersections
NOTE: mountain bikes advised

Improvements continue on this otherwise rougher leg of the SNETT, a future link in a three-state rail-trail network.

RULES & SAFETY:
   • Bicyclists should yield to pedestrians and equestrians.
   • Keep to the right, pass on the left, and alert others (*"On your left..."*) when approaching from behind.
   • Stop at road intersections and remember that drivers might not be aware of your presence.
   • Motorized vehicles are prohibited.

ORIENTATION:
Undeveloped sections of this rail-trail hold difficult riding conditions especially at the western end. Well-used, unmarked paths intertwine at points along the way so follow the rail-trail's steady line and even grade when navigating.

TRAIL DESCRIPTION:
Heading west from **Grove St.** in Franklin, the rail-trail enters woods on a relatively smooth gravel surface. It crosses **Spring St.** (0.6 miles) at a field and returns to woods on the way to **Prospect St.** (1.3 miles) where a short climb to cross the road is required at a former bridge site.

Entering Bellingham on the other side, the trail gains a smooth, stone dust surface for the next 1.6 miles. A short asphalt section eases it down a slope to **Lake St.** (1.9 miles) at another missing bridge and then rises back to the original grade on the other side. Stone dust resumes for the next mile to the crossing of **Center St.** (2.9 miles) where the trail utilizes **Fox Run Rd.** for 0.2 miles. Continuing straight where the road bends right, the last leg becomes overgrown,

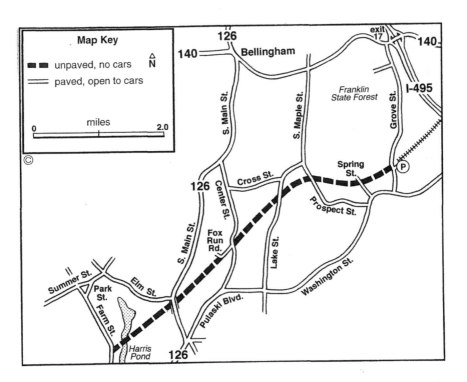

rougher with rocks and berms, and wet in a few areas. It passes under **S. Main St./Rte. 126** (4.2 miles), enters Blackstone near a view of **Harris Pond** (5.1 miles), and narrows along a fence before reaching **Farm St.** (5.3 miles).

BACKGROUND:

This route originated in 1849 as the Norfolk County Railroad and later served the New York & New England Railroad with express trains between New York and Boston. Train service along this section lasted until 1966 and the state purchased it for recreation in 1984. Future work is planned to both improve and extend the trail. Other sections of the SNETT are described in chapters 21 and 22.

DRIVING DIRECTIONS:

From I-495 take Exit 16, follow King St. (which becomes Washington St.) southwest toward Woonsocket for 1.6 miles, turn right on Grove St., and park in the lot 0.4 miles ahead on the right. The trail starts across the street.

ADDITIONAL INFORMATION:

franklinbellinghamrailtrail.org
Friends of the SNETT, facebook.com/snettfriends/

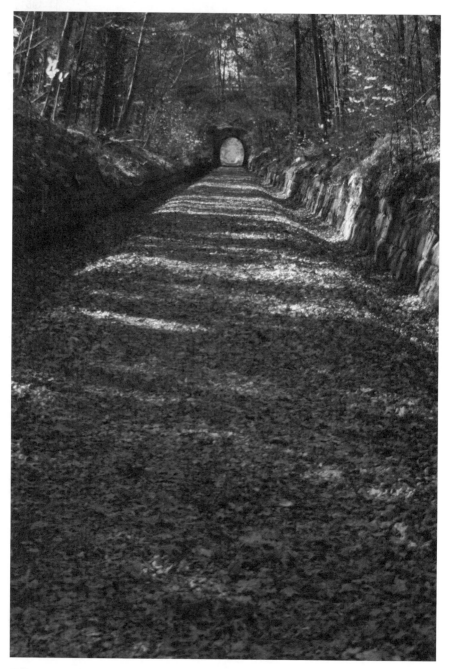

LENGTH: 14.4 miles, in several sections
SURFACE: Milford paved, Holliston & Hopkinton stone dust
TERRAIN: flat, but small slopes near Milford's Louisa Lake

This two-pronged rail-trail links Milford and Holliston with easy rolling at the headwaters of the Charles River.

RULES & SAFETY:
- Bicyclists should yield to pedestrians.
- Keep to the right, pass on the left, and alert others (*"On your left..."*) when approaching from behind.
- Dogs must be leashed and their wastes removed.
- The trail is open from one half hour before sunrise until one half hour after sunset.

ORIENTATION:
This trail exists in two sections linked by a short walk on sidewalks in downtown Milford, and scenery is equally good along both. The 4.1-mile Milford segment is entirely paved and includes a 1.4-mile detour off the rail bed which encounters small hills. The 9.2-mile Milford-Holliston branch has a paved surface for the first 2.1 miles and smooth stone dust for most of the remaining 7.1 miles.

TRAIL DESCRIPTION:
Heading north from the **E. Main St./Rte. 16** trailhead in Milford center, a paved trail follows the **Charles River** to **Fino Field**, curves left at **Milford Pond**, and reaches a T-intersection (0.3 miles) at a rail-trail. To the left (south) it lasts for only a short distance beyond E. Main St. and to the right (north) it runs for 3.8 miles to the Hopkinton town line.

Turn right and follow the rail-trail north along the pond. It intersects **Dilla St.** (1.0 mile) at a park on **Louisa Lake**, then leaves the railbed and curves through woods with small slopes for the next 1.4 miles, passing a side trail on the left along the way. After a descent to the Milford Water Co. it follows a short segment of rail bed before climbing to the edge of **Rte. 85** (2.4 miles), crossing the **exit 20** ramps for **I-495**, and passing under the highway. It returns to the rail bed and the shade of woods along the Charles River, merely

97

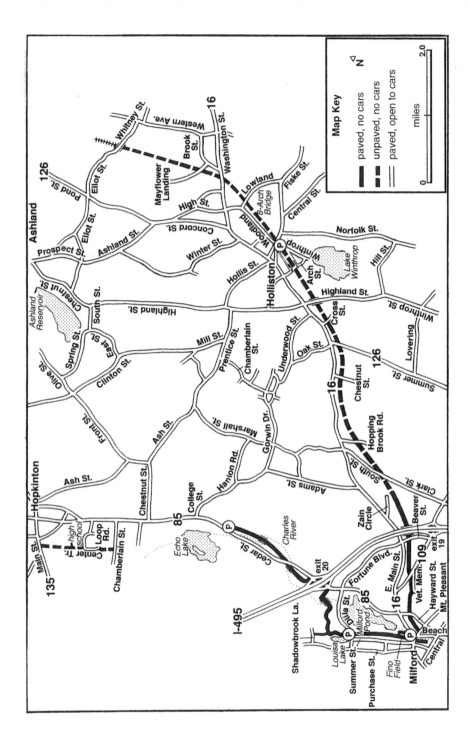

a stream at this point, and intersects Rte. 85 (3.1 miles) at a crosswalk and signal. The final mile passes wetlands, granite outcroppings, remnants of old parallel rail lines, and a second bridge over the Charles (3.5 miles) at an interpretive sign describing local railroad history. It ends at a trailhead parking lot (4.1 miles) beside Rte. 85.

A few miles north in **Hopkinton**, the mile-long **Center Tr.** utilizes another section of this rail bed with a smooth, stone dust surface and a relatively slender width through woods, adding to its natural appeal. The trail extends between **Main St./Rte. 135** near downtown Hopkinton and **Chamberlain St.** with a short interruption at **Loop Rd.** which serves nearby schools and playing fields. A side trail linking the high school intersects near the midpoint.

The southern section of the Upper Charles River Tr. is a short walk from the Main St./Rte. 16 parking lot in Milford. To reach it, cross Main St. and continue straight on the sidewalk along **Beach St.**, keep left at **Mt. Pleasant St.**, and find the bike path a short distance ahead on the left.

Heading northeast, this trail begins on a narrow corridor, widens after intersecting **Hayward St.** (0.3 miles), and curves through woods to **Veterans Memorial Dr.** (0.6 miles) where it parallels the road to the crossing of Medway Rd./Rte. 109 (0.9 miles). It continues along an open utility corridor for the next mile intersecting **Beaver St.** and passing under **I-495** (1.6 miles), then returns to the shade of woods. The asphalt surface ends just beyond **Zain Circle** (2.1 miles) and a smooth stone dust surface continues into Holliston with a slight downslope to **South St.** (2.5 miles). It extends through more woods and wetlands to **Hopping Brook Rd.** (3.1 miles), **Chestnut St.** (4.1 miles), **Summer St./Rte. 126** (4.6 miles), and **Cross St.** (5.0 miles). The trail passes through a stone arch tunnel under **Highland St.** (5.3 miles) and crosses a bridge over **Arch St.** (5.9 miles) as it approaches **Holliston** center where a small park offers greenspace and parking before **Central St.** (6.3 miles).

Crossing Central, the trail proceeds through a parking

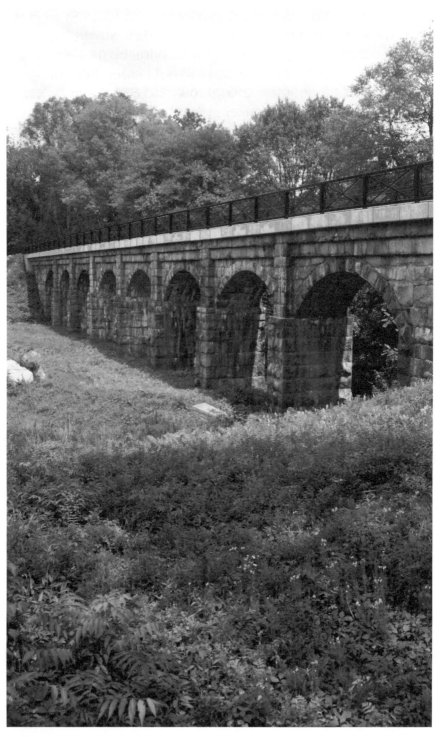

area, intersects Church St., and parallels Railroad St. and **Woodland St.** as it returns to wooded surroundings. It crosses **Bogastow Brook** on a high bridge built of eight stone arches, an impressive sight when viewed from parallel Woodland St. After intersecting **Lowland St.** (7.2 miles), the stone dust surface continues northeastward past a mix of commercial properties and natural areas, curves north across busy **Washington St./Rte. 16** (7.6 miles), and intersects **Mayflower Landing** (8.0 miles). It then enters an open wetland with interesting scenery on Dopping Brook before reaching the Sherborn town line (8.9 miles) where the finished surface ends. A rougher but rideable surface lasts to **Whitney St.** (9.2 miles).

BACKGROUND:

Most of these bike paths originated as railroads. The northern segment was constructed between Milford and Ashland in 1872 as the Hopkinton Railroad which operated until the late 1950's. The southern segment was the Milford Branch of the Boston & Worcester Railroad which opened in 1848 between Framingham and Milford and was abandoned in 1972. The first section of rail-trail was completed in Milford in 2007 and the trail has progressed in stages. Additional segments are planned to eventually create a 25-mile route through Milford, Holliston, Sherborn, Ashland, and Hopkinton.

DRIVING DIRECTIONS:

Main St./Rte. 16, Milford: From I-495 take Exit 20 and follow Rte. 85 south for 1.3 miles. Turn right on Main St./Rte. 16 west and continue for 0.4 miles, then turn right at the parking lot across from the intersection of Beach St.

Rte. 85 trailhead, Milford: From I-495 take Exit 20. Follow Rte. 85 north for 1.5 miles to the trailhead on the right.

Front St., Holliston: From I-495 take Exit 19 and follow Rte. 109 west for 1 mile. Turn right on Rte. 16 east and drive for 5.5 miles, then right on Central St. and continue for 0.3 miles. Turn right on Winthrop St. and immediately right on Front St. Park beside the trail on the right.

ADDITIONAL INFORMATION:

Friends of Holliston Trails, hollistontrails.org
Friends of the Milford Upper Charles Trail, milfordtrail.org
uppercharlestrail.org

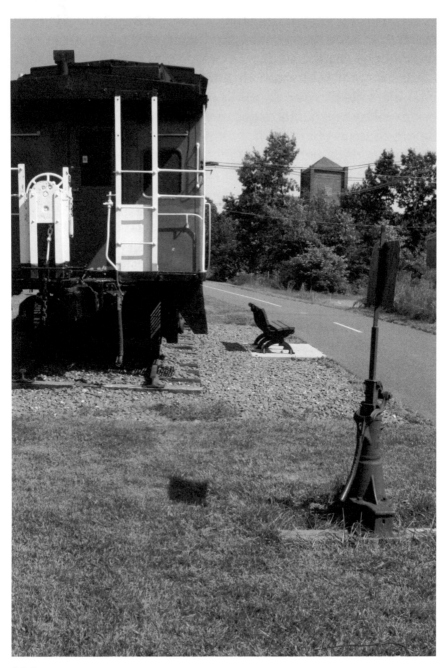

25 Assabet River Rail-Trail

Hudson-Marlborough

LENGTH: 5.3 miles
SURFACE: paved
TERRAIN: gently sloped

This two-town route mingles with the Assabet River in downtown Hudson and then climbs for several miles to neighboring Marlborough. The slope is noticeable enough to rank this rail-trail as the state's steepest.

RULES & SAFETY:
- Bicyclists should yield to pedestrians.
- Keep to the right, pass on the left, and alert others (*"On your left..."*) when approaching from behind.
- Be especially cautious in the presence of children and pets since their movements can be unpredictable.
- Do not block the trail when stopped.
- Groups should ride single-file.
- Respect nearby residents by keeping noise levels low.
- Stop at all road intersections and assume that drivers do not see you. Signs and crosswalks identify intersections and signal controls are present where necessary.
- Pets must be leashed and their wastes removed.

ORIENTATION:
The trail has a mostly north-south alignment with several trailhead parking lots along the northern end in Hudson but none at the southern end in Marlborough. The northernmost 1.5 miles of trail (to Broad St.) are generally flat while most of the remaining 3.8 miles to the south have an uphill slope toward Marlborough. Several trail kiosks offer maps with *"You are here"* designations.

TRAIL DESCRIPTION:
Begin at the northern terminus in Hudson. (Note that the sound of target shooting at a nearby gun club is frequently heard here.) Leaving the trailhead parking lot, the trail passes old bridge abutments where the Massachusetts Central Railroad once crossed overhead, continues to the intersection of **Cox St.** and **Makin St.**, then reaches **Main St./Rte. 62** (0.5 miles) at a crosswalk and signal.

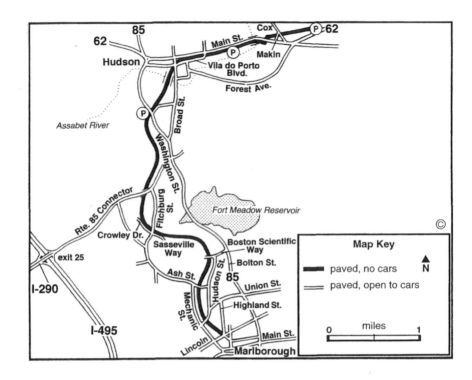

Turning right and paralleling Main St. for the next mile, the trail crosses the **Assabet River** and straightens along a grassy corridor where it passes another trailhead parking lot and a restored caboose. It narrows alongside **Vila do Porto Blvd.** (1.4 miles) as it passes close to several buildings near downtown **Hudson**, then diagonally crosses the intersection of Vila do Porto and **Broad St.** (1.5 miles). Signaled crosswalks assist trail travelers through the traffic.

Here the trail begins its climb toward Marlborough on an incline which lasts for most of the remaining 3.8 miles. Entering the shade of trees, it passes an old mill, crosses a high bridge over the Assabet River, and skirts the backyards of nearby homes before intersecting busy **Washington St./Rte.85** (2.1 miles) at a signaled crosswalk.

Woodsy surroundings take hold along the next leg to the Marlboro city line where the trail utilizes an underpass at the **Rte. 85 Connector** (3.0 miles). It descends for a short distance along **Crowley Dr.** to the intersection of **Fitchburg**

St. (3.5 miles) and then resumes an uphill angle, first beside **Sasseville Way** and then continuing into woods.

Benches offer a nice rest stop at the 4.1-mile mark where a break in the trees allows an open view of **Fort Meadow Reservoir** on the left. The trail continues across **Boston Scientific Way** (4.3 miles), **Ash St.** (4.6 miles), and **Hudson St.** (5.0 miles) before the uphill pitch finally ends and a gentle downslope relieves the last quarter-mile to the endpoint at the junction of **Lincoln St.** and **Highland St.** (5.3 miles). Continue straight on Cashman St. to follow an on-road bike route to downtown **Marlborough** only a few blocks away.

BACKGROUND:

This branch line of the Fitchburg Railroad (later the Boston & Maine) originated at S. Acton, was extended through Maynard to Gleasondale and Hudson in 1850, and reached Marlborough in 1855. After rail traffic had declined from the closing of mills and the rise of car and truck traffic, the railroad ceased operations in 1941 and the entire line had become abandoned by 1980.

A volunteer group formed in the 1990's to promote the 12-mile route's conversion to a trail and the effort eventually took hold in the five towns along the way. The Assabet River Rail-Trail officially opened in 2005 with this 5.3-mile section. With the creation of the second section in nearby Maynard and S. Acton (Chap. 26) in 2017, it is hoped that the two trails can be joined in the future. In addition, proposed construction of the Mass. Central Rail-Trail would intersect the Assabet River Rail-Trail in Hudson near the northernmost trailhead.

DRIVING DIRECTIONS:

From I-495: Take Exit 26 and follow Rte. 62 east for 4.0 miles, then look for the trailhead parking lot on the left.

From Rte. 2: Exit at Rte. 62 in Concord and drive west for 11.1 miles through Maynard and Stow and into Hudson. Look for the trailhead parking lot on the right, a half-mile past the Hudson town line.

ADDITIONAL INFORMATION:

Assabet River Rail Trail, Inc., www.arrtinc.org

26 Assabet River Rail-Trail, Assabet River N. W. R.

Maynard, Acton, Stow, Sudbury

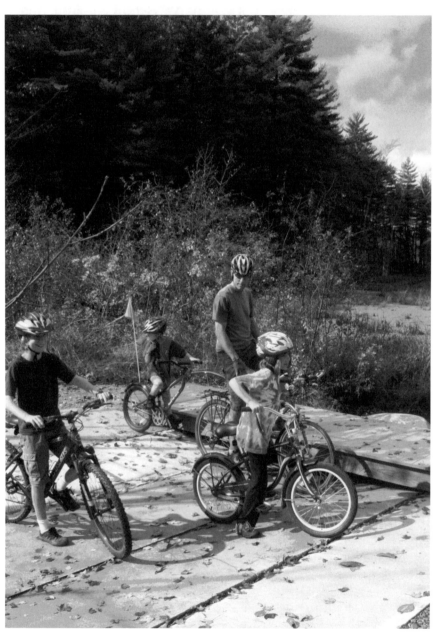

LENGTH: 3.4-mile rail-trail plus 7.4-mile network at refuge
SURFACE: rail-trail is paved, refuge has old pavement, gravel
TERRAIN: rail-trail is mostly flat, refuge has slopes
NOTE: wide-tired bikes recommended for unpaved sections

This new section of the Assabet River Rail-Trail connects downtown Maynard to both S. Acton's commuter rail station and a network of gated roads at the beautiful Assabet River National Wildlife Refuge.

RULES & SAFETY:
  • Bicyclists should yield to pedestrians.
  • Keep to the right, pass on the left, and alert others (*"On your left..."*) when approaching from behind.
  • On the rail-trail, maximum speed is 15 mph.
  • On the rail-trail, bicyclists may ride two-abreast only when it is safe to do so.
  • At the national wildlife refuge, bicycling is permitted only on designated roads (shown on the map) and is prohibited on all other routes.
  • At the national wildlife refuge, dogs are prohibited. On the rail-trail, dogs must be leashed and wastes removed.
  • At the national wildlife refuge, hunting is permitted, with the most activity occurring in the fall.
  • Watch for additional rules posted at trailheads.

ORIENTATION:
The rail-trail is accessible from trailheads at both ends, including one near the S. Acton commuter rail station. Road intersections are numerous at Maynard center but all are well-equipped with crosswalks and appropriate signage. Note that the mostly flat rail-trail holds one short, moderate slope at Summer St. in Maynard center.

The Assabet River National Wildlife Refuge roads that are designated for bicycling are identified by signs, and all other roads and trails at the refuge are closed to bicycling. Intersection numbers are displayed on the map. Several trailheads provide parking and the visitor center is equipped with water, toilets, and a wildlife exhibit.

107

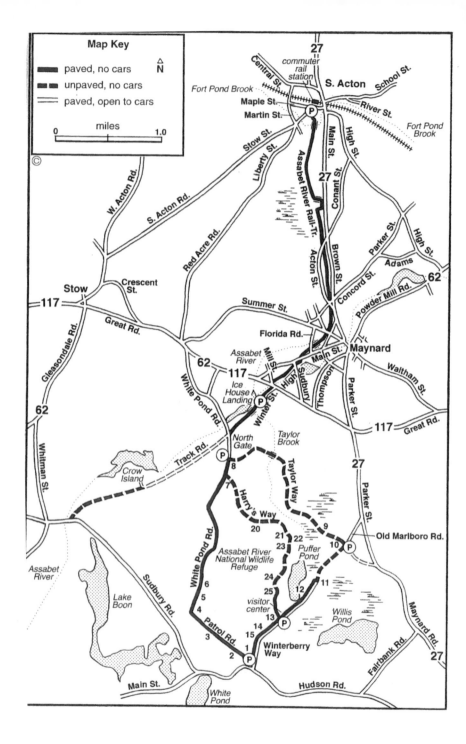

TRAIL DESCRIPTION:

Begin at the **Ice House Landing** trailhead on **Winter St.** in Maynard where a small picnic area overlooks the **Assabet River**. To the northeast (turning right on the trail when leaving the parking lot), the **Assabet River Rail-Tr.** extends for 3 miles through Maynard center to South Acton. The ride starts in woods alongside a canal which once provided water power to Maynard's nearby mills, reaches **Great Rd./Rte. 117** after a quarter-mile, and then crosses both the road and the canal to continue past homes on **High St.** Approaching downtown's commercial area, it meets a cluster of intersections at **Sudbury St.** (0.5 miles), **Main St./Rte. 62**, and **Florida Rd.** (0.8 miles), crosses a bridge over the Assabet River, and traces the edge of a parking lot up a slope to **Summer St.** (1.0 miles).

Leaving the downtown area, the trail flattens and curves northward across the triangle intersection of **Acton St.** and **Concord St.** (1.3 miles). It continues behind homes along **Rte. 27** and develops a slight downslope as it crosses Acton St. again (1.8 miles), enters Acton, and passes an open wetland. A commercial property (2.1 miles) blocks the original rail line so the trail diverts to the right alongside **Main St./Rte. 27** following boardwalks through a low-lying area back to the rail bed. The final leg descends gently through woods to a water view from a bridge over **Fort Pond Brook** (2.9 miles), turns left off the railroad grade to a trailhead parking lot, and ends at **Maple St.** (3.0 miles) opposite the **S. Acton commuter rail station**.

Heading southwest (left when facing the trail from the Winter St. parking lot) from Ice House Landing, the trail immediately crosses a bridge over **Taylor Brook** and enjoys a forested route to **White Pond Rd.** (0.4 miles) where the paved surface currently ends. Here it's possible to continue riding for 2.4 miles on unpaved rail bed along the river to **Sudbury Rd.** in Stow but bicyclists should note that part of this route, known as **Track Rd.**, accesses **Crow Island** and is open to cars, although traffic is typically light.

Nearby to the south, the 2,200-acre **Assabet River National Wildlife Refuge** holds excellent natural scenery and 7.4 miles of gated roads designated for bicycling. Surfaces are mostly unpaved and encounter moderate slopes. To find it from the rail-trail, turn left on White Pond Rd. and ride uphill away from the river for 0.2 miles to the refuge's **North Gate** trailhead at **intersection 8**. Continuing straight past the gate, a 5.6-mile perimeter loop begins with flat ground and old pavement as White Pond Rd. ventures southwest through meadows, wetlands, and eventually woods with large, earthen mounds, once World War II-era ammunition bunkers, lurking amid the trees. Turn left (southeast) at **int. 4** (1.5 miles) on **Patrol Rd.** where a straight, treeless corridor rises on a slope and reaches a trailhead parking lot (2.3 miles) at the refuge's **Hudson Rd.** entrance, then turn left on the paved bike path alongside **Winterberry Way**. It heads northeast past the **visitor center** (2.8 miles) to **int. 11** where the pavement ends and a gravel road continues downhill to a bridge between wetlands. It continues through woods to the **Old Marlboro Rd.** trailhead at **int. 10** (3.8 miles). Turn left (northwest) on 1.8-mile **Taylor Way**, another gravel road which descends to open wetland and then curves with moderate slopes through woods back to White Pond Rd. Watch for loose sand at points along this road. After crossing Taylor Brook it returns to the start of the loop at **int. 8** (5.6 miles) and North Gate.

1.8-mile **Harry's Way** bisects this peripheral route to form two 4.6-mile loop options. Beginning on the left at **int. 7** on White Pond Rd. near North Gate, this gravel road offers a woodsy, mostly uphill ride past more ammunition bunkers and several wetlands to the visitor center at **int. 13**.

BACKGROUND:

The Assabet River Rail-Tr. follows the route of the former Marlboro Branch of Fitchburg Railroad which later became part of the Boston & Maine Railroad. Built in 1850, it operated until 1941 and had become abandoned by 1980. Local rail-trail proponents organized in the 1990's and a 5.3-mile section of trail (Chap. 25) opened in Hudson and Marlboro in 2005. The 3.4-mile S. Acton and

Maynard section was completed in 2017. It is hoped that the remaining midsection can be secured to eventually reunite the line as a rail-trail.

The 2,200-acre Assabet River National Wildlife Refuge opened in 2005. Previously, the U.S. military had taken the property by eminent domain from over 100 local landowners at the onset of World War II and established the Maynard Ammunition Backup Storage Point with a network of rail lines linking 50 underground storage bunkers. Located on the Mass. Central Railroad, the depot handled supplies arriving from factories in the midwest before shipment to arsenals on the coast. After the war, the facility functioned as an annex and testing site for nearby Fort Devens.

DRIVING DIRECTIONS:

Rail-trail, Winter St. trailhead in Maynard from I-495: Take Exit 27 and follow Rte. 117 east for 7.1 miles, then turn right on Winter St. Park a quarter-mile ahead in the lot on the right.

Rail-trail, Maple St. trailhead in S. Acton from I-95: Take Exit 29B and follow Rte. 2 west for 10.5 miles, fork left at Exit 43 and follow Rte. 111 north for 0.5 miles, then turn left on Rte. 27 south and continue for 1.1 miles. After crossing a bridge over railroad tracks, turn right on Maple St. and park in the lot 0.1 miles ahead on the left.

A.R.N.W.R. Visitor Center from I-95/Rte. 128: Take Exit 26 and follow Rte. 20 west for 4.9 miles, then turn right on Rte. 27 north and drive for 3.5 miles. Where Rte. 27 turns right (just beyond Sudbury center), continue straight on Hudson Rd. for another 2.7 miles to the main entrance on the right.

A.R.N.W.R. Visitor Center from I-495: Take Exit 26 and follow Rte. 62 east for 3.5 miles to a traffic signal where Rte. 62 turns left. Continue straight on Main St. (eventually Hudson Rd.) for 3.7 miles to the main entrance on the left.

TOILETS:

A.R.N.W.R. Visitor Center

ADDITIONAL INFORMATION:

Assabet River Rail Trail, Inc., arrtinc.org
Assabet River National Wildlife Refuge, (978) 562-3527, www.fws.gov/northeast/assabetriver
Friends of Assabet River National Wildlife Refuge, farnwr.org

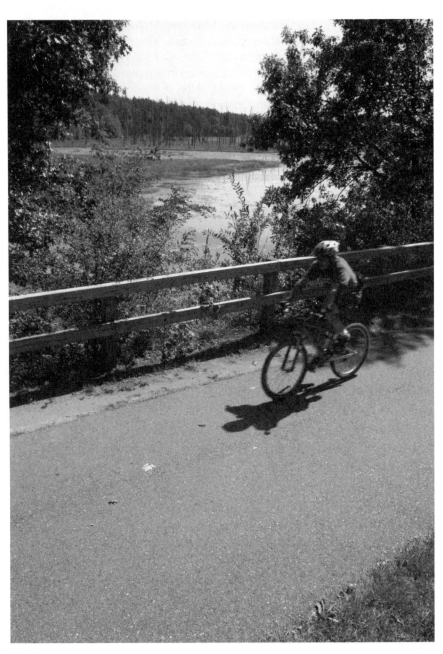

LENGTH: 12.5 miles
SURFACE: paved
TERRAIN: gentle slopes

Protected forests and farmland surround this scenic, family-friendly trail as it joins the centers of three towns.

RULES & SAFETY:
- Bicyclists should yield to pedestrians.
- Keep to the right, pass on the left, and alert others (*"On your left..."*) when approaching from behind.
- Use extra caution in the presence of children, pets, and horses since their movements can be unpredictable.
- Step off the trail when stopped so others can pass.
- Road intersections have stop signs and crosswalks. When crossing roads, assume that drivers do not see you.
- Pets must be leashed and their wastes removed.

ORIENTATION:
The trail is aligned in the north-south direction with the highest elevation at the midpoint near Groton center and the lowest elevations at the endpoints. Natural scenery is especially good along the midsection in Groton and Pepperell.

TRAIL DESCRIPTION:
Beginning at the southern endpoint at **Main St.** near the commuter rail station in downtown **Ayer**, the Nashua River Rail-Trail passes the trailhead parking lot, crosses **Groton St.**, and soon enters the shade of trees in quiet surroundings. It crosses two powerline corridors before entering Groton and straightening on a 2-mile, faint uphill slope to **Smith St.** (1.8 miles), **Peabody St.** (2.8 miles), and **Broadmeadow Rd.** (3.3 miles). The **Groton School Pond** and a vast, open wetland add interesting scenery along this stretch.

The trail skirts **Groton** center as it slips through a tunnel under **Rte. 111/Rte. 225** (3.8 miles) and crosses a bridge over **Rte. 119/Rte. 111** (4.6 miles). Farmland and forest dominate the scenery along the next mile to **Common St.** (5.1 miles) and **Sand Hill Rd.** (5.6 miles), where a small trailhead parking lot sits at the base of **Shepley Hill**.

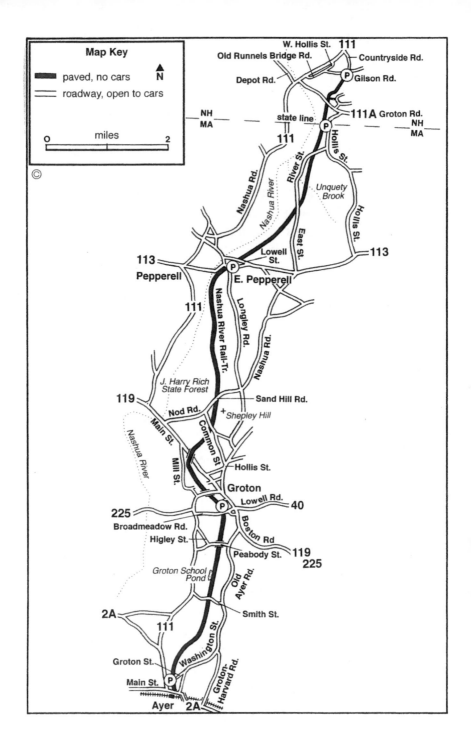

It continues beside the protected woodlands of **J. Harry Rich State Forest** where footpaths branch to the west, then enjoys water views along the **Nashua River** for the next mile to the village of **E. Pepperell**.

The trail proceeds across **Rte. 113** (8.2 miles) at a busy downtown intersection, passes another trailhead parking lot on the opposite side, and intersects **Lowell Rd.** before returning to quiet surroundings of woods, wetlands, and farmland. It enters the neighboring town of Dunstable at a powerline corridor (9.4 miles), reaches the first crossing of **River St.** (9.9 miles), then enters open scenery of wetlands along **Unquety Brook**.

The second crossing of River St. comes just before the **state line** (11.5 miles) where a side trail on the right connects a trailhead parking lot off **Hollis St.** Continuing straight, the rail-trail enters Nashua, NH and crosses **Rte. 111A** (11.9 miles), borders a residential neighborhood, and ends at another trailhead parking lot on **Gilson Rd.** (12.5 miles).

BACKGROUND:

This route originated in 1848 as the Worcester & Nashua Railroad, an important link between two growing cities. Although the line was later extended to Portland, ME, its usefulness declined in the 1900's and passenger service ended in the 1930's. Freight traffic kept the Ayer-Pepperell stretch in operation until 1982.

Massachusetts purchased its portion of the line in 1987 and developed it as a recreational trail in 2002. New Hampshire extended the trail north to Gilson Rd. in 2006.

DRIVING DIRECTIONS:

Ayer trailhead from I-495: Take Exit 30 and follow Rte. 2A west for 5.6 miles. Just after downtown Ayer, turn right on Groton St. and park in the lot immediately on the right.

Nashua trailhead from Rte. 3 (Everett Tpke.): Take Exit 5W and follow Rte. 111 west for 3 miles. Turn left on Countyside Dr. and continue for 0.3 miles to the end, then cross Gilson Rd. to enter the trailhead parking lot.

TOILETS:

Ayer trailhead

ADDITIONAL INFORMATION:

Willard Brook State Forest, (978) 597-8802

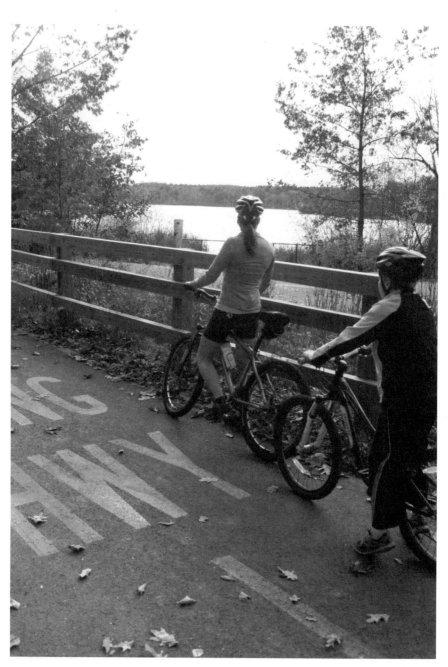

LENGTH: 11.7 miles, plus 3.8 miles under construction
SURFACE: paved
TERRAIN: slight slopes

Growing in both length and popularity, the Bruce Freeman is destined to connect Lowell and Framingham with car-free commuting and recreation. The trail's newly-created Acton section is a highlight for natural scenery.

RULES & SAFETY:
- Bicyclists should yield to pedestrians.
- Keep to the right, pass on the left, and alert others (*"On our left..."*) when approaching from behind.
- Use extra caution in the presence of children and pets since their movements can be unpredictable.
- Stop at road intersections and assume that drivers do not see you.
- Step off the trail when stopped so others can pass.
- Sections of trail that are under construction are closed to use, as posted by signs.
- Park only in designated locations.
- Dogs must be leashed and their wastes removed.
- Watch for additional regulations posted at trailheads.

ORIENTATION:
Trailhead parking lots are provided in Acton and Chelmsford. Road intersections are equipped with stop signs, crosswalks, posted street names, and signal controls where necessary. The trail also offers mileage markers, benches, and portable toilets (in season) at several locations. Natural scenery is best south of Chelmsford center and especially good in Acton where the trail mingles with Nashoba Brook and surrounding wetlands. Elevation changes are minimal but the midsection near Rte. 225 is the trail's highest point and the ends are low points.

Construction is underway to extend the trail south into Concord, connecting the West Concord commuter rail station along the way. Until trail construction is completed, this section is not open for use.

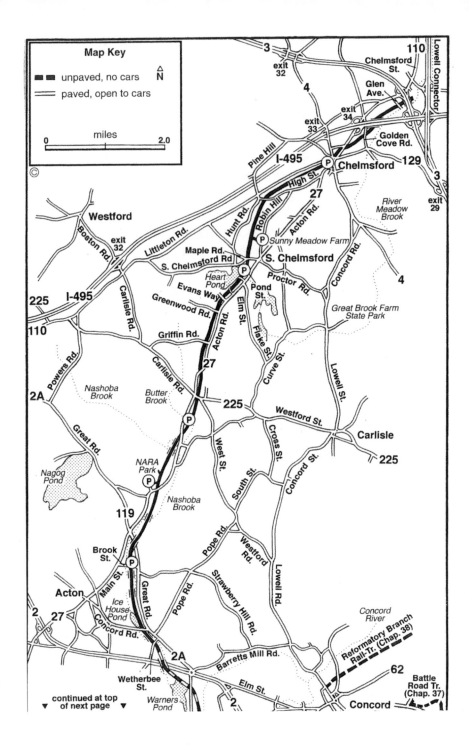

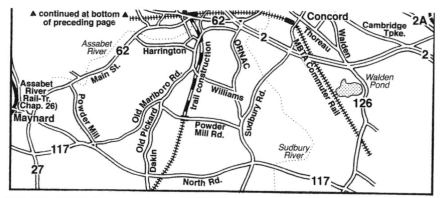

TRAIL DESCRIPTION:

Begin at **Brook St.** where trailhead parking is provided behind the Gould Plaza shopping center on **Rte. 2A/119**. To the south (turning left on the trail and crossing Brook St.), the Bruce Freeman Rail-Trail extends for 1.5 miles through a mix of natural surroundings and commercial areas. Following **Nashoba Brook** downstream and crossing it at 3 points, this section passes **Ice House Pond**, intersects **Concord Rd.** (1.2 miles) and **Wetherbee St.** (1.4 miles), then dead-ends at a set of benches (1.5 miles) a short distance before **Rte. 2**. Future construction will extend the trail over the highway and into Concord.

To the north (turning right on the trail from Gould Plaza), the Bruce Freeman Rail-Trail extends for 10.2 miles. Heading upstream along Nashoba Brook, it rises on a curved bridge spanning **Rte. 2A/119** (0.3 miles) and descends into conservation land on the other side, crosses a bridge over the brook, and passes stone foundations of the 1800's Ebenezer Wood Pencil Factory.

Ahead, the crosswalk at **Main St./Rte. 27** (1.4 miles) has the assistance of a flashing signal. This is the first of five intersections equipped with flashing signals along the next 3 miles of trail, and each location involves fast-moving traffic and limited visibility so use caution when crossing.

The Bruce Freeman detours from the rail bed at **NARA Park** (1.6 miles), also known as Nathaniel Allen

Recreation Area, where toilets, drinking water, and parking are provided. The trail joins a walking path for a short distance along the edge of a pond and circles a lumber business before returning to the rail line (2.0 miles).

Next it intersects the access road for the Nashoba Sportsmens Club (2.3 miles) where gunshots from target shooting are sometimes heard. It crosses a bridge over **Nashoba Brook** at the confluence of **Butter Brook** in an area of open wetlands, crosses Main St./Rte. 27 (2.7 miles) again, and passes a trailhead parking lot (3.0 miles) near the Carlisle town line. After only a few hundred feet the trail continues into Westford and meets **Carlisle Rd./Rte. 225** (3.4 miles) at a traffic signal. It parallels **Acton Rd./Rte. 27** before crossing the roadway (3.9 miles) a final time at an S-curve with limited visibility, so use caution when crossing.

The slight upward pitch levels at the trail's high point near **Griffin Rd.** (4.3 miles) and a slight downslope begins. Continuing along Rte. 27 behind a buffer of trees, the trail crosses the Chelmsford town line at **Greenwood Rd.** (4.9 miles), intersects **Evans Way** (5.1 miles), and enjoys a glimpse of **Heart Pond** on the left. A cluster of shoreline homes borders the next half-mile before the trail joins the water's edge and intersects **Pond St.** (5.8 miles) at a trailhead parking lot and local beach.

It crosses **Maple Rd.** (6.0 miles) near the village of **S. Chelmsford** and continues past conservation land to a set of powerlines (6.4 miles) where a side trail leads to the **Sunny Meadow Farm** trailhead. Curving northeast, the trail crosses **High St.** (7.1 miles) and follows Beaver Brook downstream through conservation land to Cushing Plaza (8.4 miles) where it emerges from woods at the edge of a parking lot in **Chelmsford center**.

At the edge of Rte. 4/110, the trail utilizes sidewalks and a signaled crosswalk in order to cross a busy intersection. Wood fencing guides it through a commercial area to the intersection of **Chelmsford St./Rte. 110** at Fletcher Rd. (8.8 miles) where the trail again relies on sidewalks for a short distance along both sides of the road. Returning to woods, it approaches the sound of **I-495** at ramps for **exit 34**, intersects **Golden Cove Rd.** (9.3 miles), and proceeds under highway bridges (9.5 miles). The final leg passes behind shopping centers and industrial buildings on the way to **Glen Ave.** (10.0 miles), follows **River Meadow Brook** for a short distance, and enters a lighted tunnel under **Rte. 3** (10.2 miles). The trail ends on the other side at a parking lot for an office tower off Chelmsford St./Rte. 110 where limited trailhead parking is allowed on weekends and holidays.

BACKGROUND:

This route originated in 1871 as the Framingham & Lowell Railroad. When train service stopped in 1982 Bruce Freeman, rail-trail enthusiast and state representative from Chelmsford, proposed that the state-owned rail line be converted to a bike path for all to enjoy. The trail project was named posthumously in his honor and slowly took hold with the first 6.8-mile section in Chelmsford and Westford built in 2008 and a 4.9-mile extension south to Acton opened in 2018. The trail will reach Concord soon with an additional 3.8 miles under construction, and design work is in progress southward in Sudbury across the Mass. Central Railroad, another potential rail-trail. The Bruce Freeman is envisioned to link Framingham in the south and Lowell in the north, a 25-mile distance.

DRIVING DIRECTIONS:

Gould Plaza from I-95/Rte. 128: Take Exit 29B and follow Rte. 2 west for 8.1 miles to the Concord rotary. Continue west on Rte. 2A for 2.2 miles, turn left on Brook St., and park in the lot on the right, behind the shopping center.

Cushing Plaza from I-495: Take Exit 34 and follow Rte. 110 west for 0.7 miles. After Rte. 110 turns right at Rte. 4 in downtown Chelmsford, turn immediately left into a long, narrow parking lot and park at the end beside the trail. More parking is available across the street behind Old Town Hall.

TOILETS:

Chelmsford at Cushing Plaza and Pond St., Acton at NARA Park

ADDITIONAL INFORMATION:

Friends of the Bruce Freemain Rail Trail, brucefreemanrailtrail.org

29 Methuen Rail-Trail
Lawrence-Salem, NH

LENGTH: 3.1 miles
SURFACE: gravel, processed stone, recycled asphalt
TERRAIN: flat
NOTE: wide-tired bicycles recommended

This simple, coarsely surfaced rail bed is one of the first legs of a future long-distance trail linking Methuen and Lawrence to Manchester, NH and beyond.

RULES & SAFETY:
- Bicyclists should yield to pedestrians.
- Keep to the right, pass on the left, and alert others (*"On your left..."*) when approaching from behind.
- Crosswalks are not present so stop at road intersections and remember that drivers might not see you.
- Pets must be leashed and their wastes removed.
- Watch for additional information posted at trailheads.

ORIENTATION:

The trail has a north-south alignment with a trailhead at Methuen center near the midpoint. Road intersections are few but, as a result of the trail's relatively undeveloped condition, currently do not have crosswalks, signs, and other safety features. Continuing north into New Hampshire, the Salem Rail-Trail remains unfinished and eventually contends with high traffic areas which are currently inadvisable for trail usage.

TRAIL DESCRIPTION:

Heading south from the **Methuen center** trailhead (turning right when facing the trail from the road), the trail parallels **Railroad St.** past the former train station, across **Union St.**, under **Oakland Ave.** (0.3 miles), and along a leafy corridor above the **Spicket River**. After a half-mile a view of the river and mills of **Lawrence** opens on the left as the trail crosses the city line on an elevated grade and then

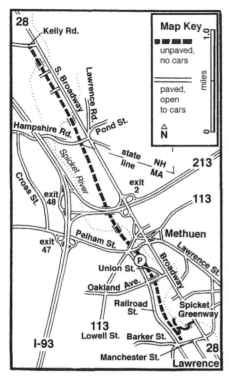

ends before a bridge over **Manchester St.** (1.0 mile).

Turn hard left at the end of a chainlink fence to follow the **Spicket Greenway**, a paved trail which descends to a playground, passes old mill buildings, and crosses a bridge over the river to reach **Broadway/Rte. 28.**

Heading north from the Methuen center trailhead (turning left when facing the trail from the road), the trail passes under a broad bridge for **Lowell St./Rte. 113** and Osgood St. and soon crosses the **Spicket River** at the Nevins Bird Sanctuary. It passes under bridges for **Rte. 213** (0.6 miles) and straightens along a line of utility poles to the state line where it enters Salem, NH as the **Salem Rail-Trail**. Crossing **Hampshire Rd.** (1.3 miles), it continues into a commercial area along **S. Broadway/Rte. 28**, crossing the Spicket River again before reaching **Kelly Rd.** (2.4 miles). Cycling is not recommended north of this point as conditions degrade with rougher surfaces and a lack of safe crossing points at busy intersections.

BACKGROUND:

This route originated in 1849 as the Manchester & Lawrence Railroad and operated until the 1980's. It was transformed to a trail in 2012 through the Iron Horse Preservation Society which removed the rails and ties and applied the surface material. Other sections of this line in Windham, Derry, and Londonderry, NH are also rail-trails.

DRIVING DIRECTIONS:

From I-93: Take Exit 47 and follow Pelham St. east for 0.7 miles to a traffic signal. Turn right on Railroad St. and park in the lot 0.1 miles ahead on the left, next to the trail.

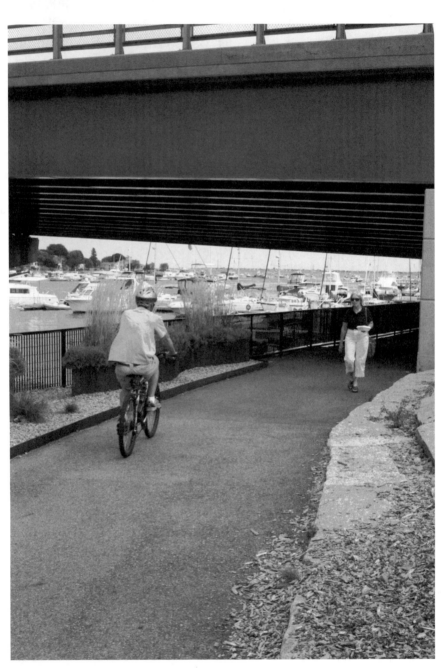

LENGTH: 9.4 miles, plus 1.2 miles under construction
SURFACE: mostly paved, some processed stone
TERRAIN: mild slopes

Joining 3 towns, the expanding Coastal Trails Network is improving car-free connections to the area's commercial centers as well as its excellent natural scenery.

RULES & SAFETY:
  • Bike paths under construction are not open to use.
  • Bicyclists should yield to pedestrians.
  • Keep to the right, pass on the left, and alert others (*"On your left..."*) when approaching from behind.
  • Step off the trail when stopped so others can pass.
  • Dogs must be leashed and their wastes removed.

ORIENTATION:
Several trail segments are separated by short, on-road detours but future construction will provide improved connections. The Eastern Marsh Tr. and the Clipper City Rail-Tr. offer the most interesting scenery while the Ghost Tr. and the Riverwalk explore mostly wooded areas.

TRAIL DESCRIPTION:
Salisbury's 1.7-mile **Ghost Tr.** extends east from a trailhead on **Rabbit Rd.** with a smooth surface of processed stone. It begins in open surroundings beside a solar energy site and enters woods for the remaining distance, crossing **Bartlett St.** and **Cushing St.** before ending at **Lion's Park**.

The 1.8-mile **Garrison Tr.** begins nearby heading south from **Rte. 110** alongside **I-95**, crossing the **Merrimack River** on the **Whittier Bridge** into Newburyport, accessing **Ferry Rd.**, and ending at a commuter parking lot on **Storey Ave.** Across the street, the 1.2-mile **Gloria Braumhardt Bike Path** continues south following an abandoned roadway through a natural area to **Hale St.**

Extending west from the Ghost Tr. at Rabbit Rd., a half-mile of trail will be constructed to pass under I-95 and connect the 1.4-mile **Amesbury Riverwalk** at the **Carriage Town Marketplace**. The Riverwalk currently starts behind

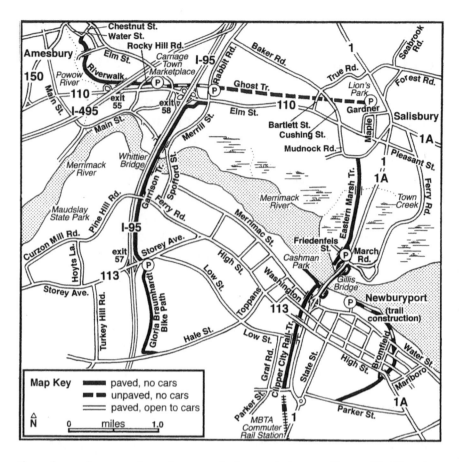

the shopping center, descends to an intersection with **Rocky Hill Rd.**, passes under **I-495**, curves north along the **Powow River**, and ends at **Water St.** near downtown **Amesbury**.

The 1.4-mile **Eastern Marsh Tr.** offers the area's best views. To find it from the east end of the Ghost Tr. at Lion's Park exit on Lions Way, turn left on **Gardner**, right on **Maple**, left on **Elm St./Rte. 110**, then immediately right on **Mudnock Rd.** Starting a third of a mile ahead on the left, the Eastern Marsh Tr. emerges from treecover heading south across a vast saltmarsh surrounding **Town Creek**, then returns to woods for the last half-mile to an overlook on the Merrimack.

A side trail links downtown Newburyport. Descending to cross **Friedenfels St.**, it circles under the **Gillis Bridge** and returns to a sidewalk on the eastern side of Rte. 1 where cyclists can walk the quarter-mile span over the **Merrimack River** enjoying a harbor view along the way. On the other side, turn left on a path descending under the bridge to join the 1.1-mile **Clipper City Rail-Tr.** which continues south to **Parker St.** and the **MBTA commuter rail station** It begins with an uphill to a bridge over **Merrimac St.**, intersects **Washington St.**, passes under **High St.** beside massive retaining walls, and enjoys an area of sculptures as it spans **Low St.** A half-mile to the east, another 0.8-mile leg of the Clipper City Rail-Tr. extends from Parker St. north to **Water St.** and a view of the Merrimack River Estuary, with another 0.7 miles under construction along the downtown riverfront.

BACKGROUND:

The Clipper City Rail-Tr. and Eastern Marsh Tr. follow the former Eastern Railroad, built in 1840 from Boston to Portsmouth, NH. The Amesbury Riverwalk and Ghost Tr. follow the Eastern's Amesbury Branch, built in 1848 for the town's carriage and sleigh manufacturing industry. These products were draped with white cloth during shipment, lending the name "ghost trains."

Trail construction began in 2001 with Amesbury's Riverwalk and has continued in phases. Current construction projects include the Clipper City extension along Newburyport's waterfront and a connection between the Ghost Tr. and Amesbury's Riverwalk.

Future construction will extend the Clipper City Rail-Tr. south and the Eastern Marsh Tr. north as part of the Border-to-Boston Tr. (Chap. 31). This will also serve the East Coast Greenway, a planned route between Maine and Florida.

DRIVING DIRECTIONS:

• **Ghost Tr. from I-95:** Take Exit 58A and follow Rte. 110 east to the first traffic signal. Turn left on Rabbit Rd. and look for the trailhead a short distance ahead on the right.

• **Old Eastern Marsh Tr. from I-95:** Take Exit 57 and follow Rte. 113 east for 2.3 miles. Following signs for Rte. 1 north, turn left on Summer St., merge onto Rte. 1, cross the river, turn left on Friedenfels St., and park on the right.

• **Riverwalk Tr. from I-95:** Take Exit 58B and follow Rte. 110 west for 0.3 miles. Turn right to enter the Carriage Town Marketplace, circle to the left, and park beside the trail.

ADDITIONAL INFORMATION:

Coastal Trails Coalition, coastaltrails.org

31 Border-to-Boston Tr.
Peabody-Boxford

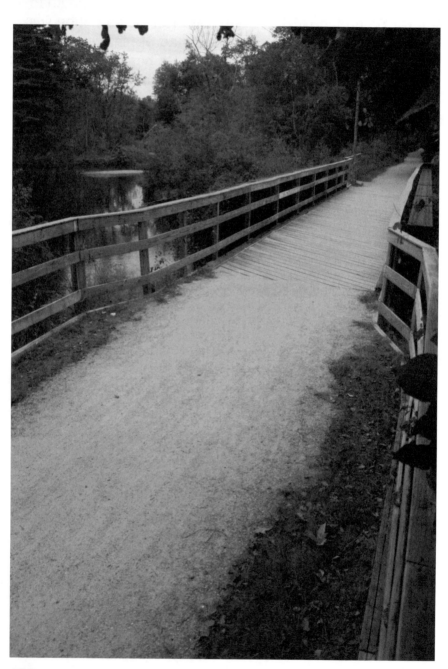

LENGTH: 10.9 miles
SURFACE: stone dust aggregate
TERRAIN: slight slopes

A rail-trail destined to join the outskirts of Boston with New Hampshire and Maine, the "B2B" visits the centers of Danvers and Topsfield and beautiful scenery in between.

RULES & SAFETY:
· Bicyclists should yield to pedestrians.
· Keep to the right, pass on the left, and alert others (*"On your left..."*) when approaching from behind.
· Step off the trail when stopped so others can pass.
· Dogs must be leashed and their wastes removed.
· The trail is open from dawn to dusk.

ORIENTATION:
The trail's north-south alignment spans the towns of Peabody, Danvers, Wenham, Topsfield, and Boxford with town lines posted at each border. In Danvers, signs display intersecting street names and trail mileages at 0.1-mile intervals. Natural scenery is especially good in Wenham and Topsfield where river and wetland views are plentiful.

TRAIL DESCRIPTION:
Heading south (right when facing the trail) from the **Hobart St.** parking lot in **Danvers**, the trail extends for 2.6 miles. It contends with frequent intersections until **Collins St.** (1.1 miles), passes a commercial area before crossing a bridge over **Andover St/Rte. 114** (1.7 miles), and enters Peabody where an incline develops amid woods and stone walls. The trail ends at **Lowell St.** (2.6 miles) and an **I-95** underpass near the **Independence Greenway** (Chap. 32).

Heading north (left when facing the trail) from Hobart St. in Danvers, the trail extends for 8.3 miles. A cluster of road intersections including busy **Maple St./Rte 35** (0.2 miles) slow the first half-mile then a mile-long incline carries the trail through residential neighborhoods to **Wenham St.** (1.5 miles). Woods take hold as it descends through a bedrock cut into Wenham (2.4 miles), then a vast wetland

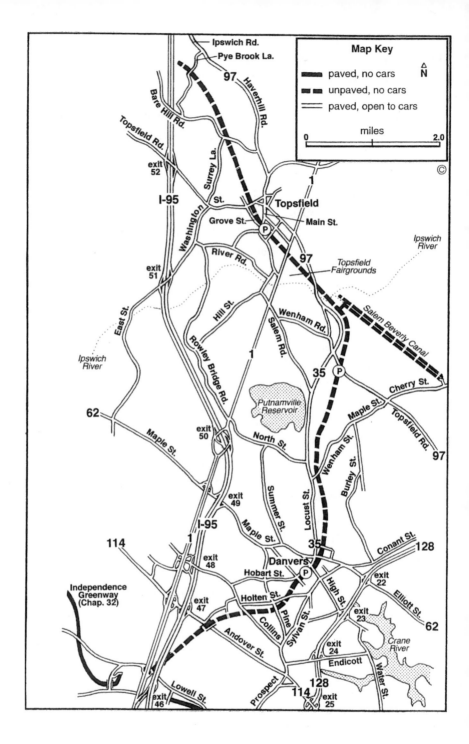

opens the view near **Putnamville Reservoir**.

The trail intersects **Topsfield Rd./Rte. 97** (3.1 miles) at a parking area and signaled crosswalk, straightens across another wetland, and curves northwest at the Topsfield line (3.7 miles). Watch for a trail on the right linking the **Salem Beverly Canal**, a 1.9-mile-long water supply channel with paths on both sides and a connection to **Cherry St.** The rail-trail continues over the **Ipswich River** (4.3 miles), crosses Rte. 97 (4.5 miles), and passes the open area of the **Topsfield Fairgrounds**. Just ahead, the crossing of **Rte. 1** (5.1 miles) deserves caution since traffic speeds are high.

The trail reaches **Topsfield** center at a parking lot before **Main St.** (5.6 miles) and continues past a shopping center. North of **Washington St.** (5.9 miles) the treadway narrows to a smooth, earthen path and straightens between borders of mowed grass, dipping to the intersection of **Bare Hill Rd.** (7.0 miles) at a missing bridge and then hitting the Boxford town line (7.6 miles). The trail intersects **Pye Brook La.** (8.1 miles) and dead-ends before **I-95** (8.3 miles).

BACKGROUND:

The Danvers & Georgetown Railroad, later known as the Newburyport Branch of the Boston & Maine, was built in 1854 and operated until 1977. Now owned by the MBTA and National Grid, the right of way has been transformed to a trail through local efforts that have progressed in stages. Together with the nearby Independence Greenway (Chapter 32), the Border-to-Boston Tr. is part of the East Coast Greenway from Maine to Florida.

DRIVING DIRECTIONS:

• **Danvers from Rte. 128:** Take Exit 23 and follow Rte. 35 north for 0.8 miles. Turn left on Hobart St. and look for the parking lot 0.1 miles ahead on the left.

• **Topsfield from I-95:** Take Exit 52 and follow Topsfield Rd. east for 0.8 miles. Keep left on Washington St. and drive for 0.6 miles, then fork right on High St. Ext. At the end turn right (south) on Main St. and continue for a quarter-mile, turn left on Park St., and then right at the parking lot.

ADDITIONAL INFORMATION:

Topsfield Linear Common, friendsoftopsfieldtrails.org
Danvers Rail Trail, danversrailtrail.org

32 Independence Greenway
Peabody

LENGTH: 4.7 miles in 2 parts, plus 1.5 miles on-road
SURFACE: paved
TERRAIN: flat

This two-part rail-trail is a worthy escape route from busy highways but its on-road midsection is to be avoided.
RULES & SAFETY:
- Bicyclists should yield to pedestrians.
- Keep to the right, pass on the left, and alert others ("On your left...") when approaching from behind.
- Blasting at a nearby quarry occasionally closes the trail near Russell St. for 10-minute periods, as posted.
- Dogs must be leashed and their wastes removed.

ORIENTATION:
The 3-mile western leg has excellent natural scenery while the 1.7-mile eastern leg traverses a more developed area and accesses the Northshore Mall at Rte. 128. The 1.5-mile on-road midsection involves a relatively high level of car traffic but passes the Border-to-Boston Tr. (Chap. 31).

TRAIL DESCRIPTION:
Beginning at the **Northshore Mall**, the trail's first leg quickly departs the noise of **Rte. 128**. It crosses the junction of **Lowell St.** and **Prospect St.** (0.5 miles), parallels Lowell St. and natural scenery along **Proctor Brook**, then ends at **Peabody Rd.** (1.7 miles) where a 1.5-mile on-road detour starts right. Turn left on Lowell St., pass under **I-95** at the **Border-to-Boston Tr.** (Chap. 31), under **Rte. 1**, fork left on **Johnson St.** (2.7 miles), then turn left at **Lt. Ross Park**. Keep right at the bottom (3.2 miles) for the trail's next leg.

The second leg curves north through open wetlands, intersects Lowell St. (3.9 miles) and **Russell St.** (4.3 miles), then passes a **quarry** where 10 minute-periods of blasting occasionally close the trail, as posted. The last stretch turns

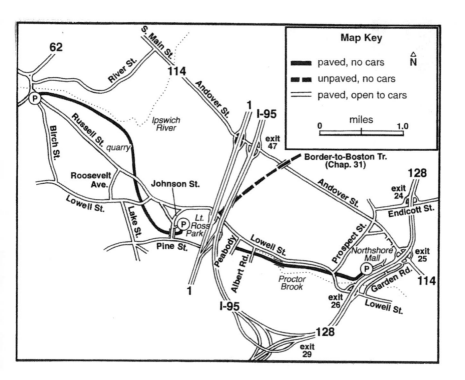

west alongside the **Ipswich River** to Russell St. (6.2 miles).

BACKGROUND:

The Independence Greenway follows the former Salem & Lowell Railroad which was completed in 1850. Train service ended in the 1980's, proposals for a rail-trail arose in the 1990's, and construction started in 2008. A link in the East Coast Greenway, it is envisioned to eventually extend east to Salem and west to Tewksbury.

DRIVING DIRECTIONS:

Northshore Mall from Rte. 128 northbound: Take Exit 25A, turn right off the ramp, take the first right and pass under the highway, then turn left with Essex Ctr. Dr. Park in the lot straight ahead where the road turns hard right.

Northshore Mall from Rte. 128 southbound: Take Exit 25B for Rte. 114 west, turn left into the mall entrance, then turn left and follow the perimeter road alongside the highway. Park straight ahead where the road turns right.

Lt. Ross Park: From Rte. 128 take Exit 26 and follow Lowell St. west for 2.5 miles. Fork left on Johnson St. and drive for 0.4 miles, then turn left at the park entrance.

33 Marblehead Rail-Trail Salem Bike Path

Marblehead, Salem, Swampscott

LENGTH: 4 miles
SURFACE: mostly stone dust/aggregate, limited pavement
TERRAIN: flat

Marblehead has four miles of freedom in its quiet rail-trail, a welcome alternative to the area's cramped streets.

RULES & SAFETY:
- Bicyclists should yield to pedestrians.
- Keep to the right, pass on the left, and alert others (*"On your left..."*) when approaching from behind.
- Respect nearby residents by keeping noise levels low.
- Crosswalks and gates identify trail/road intersections. Stop before crossing and assume that drivers do not see you.
- Pets must be leashed and their wastes removed.

ORIENTATION:
The rail-trail splits in two directions near the Bessom St. trailhead. The Salem Branch forks right (west) through woodsy, natural areas and links the short, paved Salem Bike Path. The Swampscott Branch forks left (southwest) through residential surroundings with numerous street crossings.

TRAIL DESCRIPTION:
The rail-trail leaves the **Bessom St.** parking lot heading west, passing under a bridge for **Village St.** and rising to a fenced utility yard where it forks after 0.2 miles.

Heading right, the Salem Branch passes the **Hawthorn Pond Conservation Area**, crosses **West Shore Dr.** (0.8 miles from Bessom St.), then enters the **Wyman Woods Conservation Area**. It reaches the Salem border at a view of **Salem Harbor** and continues across busy **Rte. 114** (1.5 miles) as the **Salem Bike Path**, a paved trail to **Rte. 1A** and **Canal St.** (2.2 miles). Construction will soon extend the trail north for another 1.5 miles to downtown Salem.

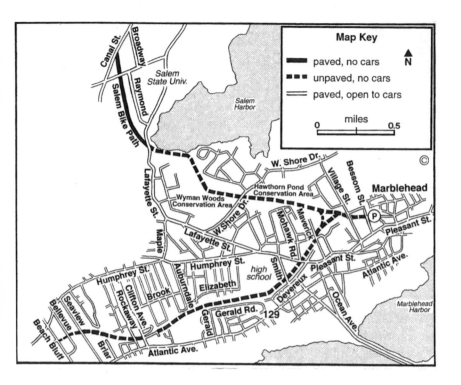

The 1.9-mile Swampscott Branch heads southwest crossing 3 roads in the first half-mile including **Pleasant St./Rte. 114.** Straightening, it continues past playing fields and residential neighborhoods for the next mile, utilizes a paved parking lot and access road before **Clifton Ave.** (1.5 miles), and passes Ware Pond Conservation Area. The trail enters Swampscott after **Seaview Ave.** (1.8 miles) and ends nearby at **Beach Bluff Ave.**

BACKGROUND:

The trail follows two segments of the former Eastern Railroad. The first, completed in 1839, runs west from Marblehead to Salem and the second, completed in 1873, runs southwest to Swampscott. After train service ended in 1959, the route eventually gained new value for the town as both a utility corridor and recreational trail.

DRIVING DIRECTIONS:

From I-95/Rte. 128 take Exit 25A. Follow Rte. 114 east for 6 miles to its endpoint at Rte. 129, continue straight on Pleasant St. for a half-mile, then turn left on Bessom St. and park in the public lot on the right, across from the trail.

LENGTH: 2.5 miles
SURFACE: paved
TERRAIN: flat

Complementing a popular beach, this short bike path enjoys an oceanfront location and no road intersections.

RULES & SAFETY:

• Bicyclists should yield to pedestrians.

• During swimming season, watch for visitors crossing as they travel between the beach and parking lots.

• Keep to the right, pass on the left, and alert others (*"On your left..."*) when approaching from behind.

• Dogs must be leashed and their wastes removed, and dogs are not allowed on the beach from May 1 - Sept. 30.

• Note that the area is exposed to wind and weather.

ORIENTATION:

The trail's waterfront location and lack of intersections make it difficult to get lost. Expansive parking stretches along the beach providing many options for trail access.

TRAIL DESCRIPTION:

Beginning at **Main Gate** in Nahant at the south end, the paved pathway heads north paralleling **Nahant Beach Pkwy.** on a narrow spit of land connecting Nahant to the mainland at Lynn. Dunes separate the broad beach which arcs to the right far into the distance around **Nahant Bay**.

The trail passes the **Ward Bath House** (1.2 miles) at the midpoint. The reservation's headquarters, a first aid station, and toilet facilities are located inside the building which is open only during the swimming season.

The path changes noticeably at this point, switching from asphalt to concrete and leaving the open dunes of the peninsula to join a seawall built along **Lynn Shore Dr.** where handsome homes overlook the bay. It follows the curve of

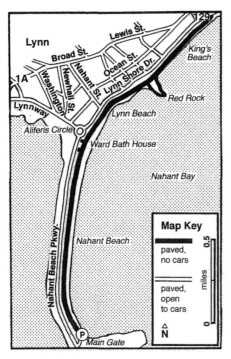

Lynn Beach for the next half-mile with steps descending to the sand at points along the way, but note that waves can spray onto the path at high tide during rough conditions.

A side trail loops through **Red Rock**, a small point of land formed by volcanic activity 500 million years ago, and benches offer a place to rest with a nice view.

The path's final stretch follows a seawall past **King's Beach**, enters Swampscott, and joins the edge of Humphrey St./**Rte. 129**. The endpoint (2.5 miles) offers a high-ground view over the water to the Nahant peninsula, the entire beach reservation, and the skyline of Boston.

BACKGROUND:

Originated in 1855, this was one of the Boston area's first public beaches. The surrounding reservation was established in the 1890's as part of an effort to encircle Boston with greenspace and parkways. Its paved trail was built in the 1980's and will eventually link the nearby Northern Strand Community Tr. (Chap. 42) which extends from Lynn southwest to Everett and the Mystic River.

DRIVING DIRECTIONS:

From I-95/Rte. 128: Take Exit 44 and follow Rte. 1 south for a short distance, then follow Rte. 129 east for 3.6 miles. Fork left on Rte. 129A and drive for 2.5 miles, then turn right on Lynn Shore Dr. and continue for 1 mile to a rotary. Following signs to Nahant, take Nahant Beach Pkwy. to the end of the median and turn left to enter the parking lot. (Cars enter at the beach's south end and exit at the north.)

TOILETS:

Ward Bath House during swimming season

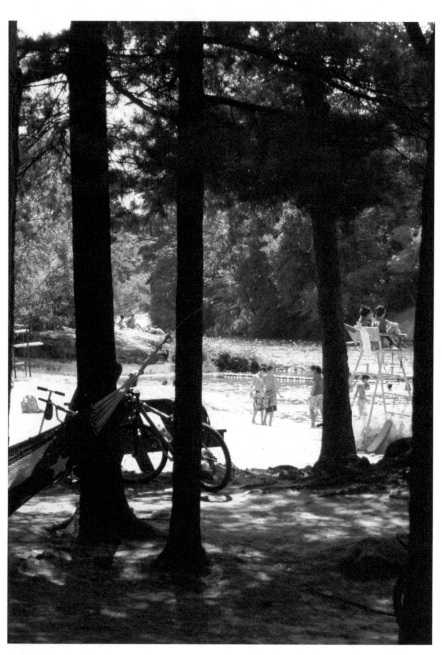

LENGTH: 3.7 miles
SURFACE: paved
TERRAIN: hilly

In summer, combine a ride at this gated road network with a swim and picnic at Breakheart's sandy beach. The reservation's quiet woodlands include a hilly terrain of boulders and ledge, providing plenty of challenge for cyclists and other exercisers.

RULES & SAFETY:

- Bicyclists should yield to pedestrians.
- Steep grades, sharp corners, and two-way traffic warrant caution. Ride at a safe speed, keep to the right, pass on the left, and alert others (*"On your left..."*) when approaching from behind.
- Use extra caution in the presence of children and pets since their movements can be unpredictable.
- Step off the trail when stopped so others can pass.
- Bicycling is not permitted on single-track trails.
- Pets must be leashed and their wastes removed.
- Swimming is permitted only in the supervised area.
- First aid is available at the swimming beach in season.
- The reservation closes at sunset each day.
- Watch for additional information posted at trailheads.

ORIENTATION:

Two trailheads access the reservation. The main entrance offers a visitor center at the southeast corner of the trail system in Saugus while the Hemlock Rd. parking area is located at the northwest corner in Wakefield and offers closer access to the swimming beach but no conveniences. A gated network of paved roads forms two loops between these parking lots.

The beach is the reservation's primary attraction in summer during the swimming season and bicyclists should expect to encounter high visitation on fairweather days. Breakheart also offers hiking trails (closed to bicycling) which climb to hilltops for views of Boston and the ocean.

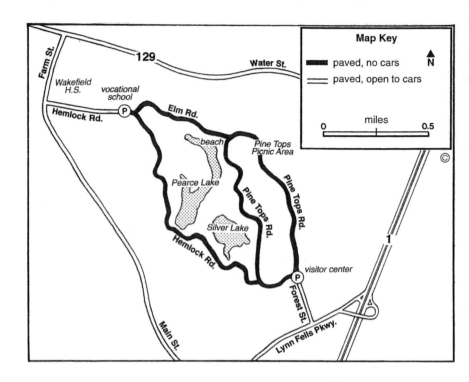

TRAIL DESCRIPTION:

Begin at the **visitor center** trailhead at the end of **Forest St.** in Saugus where **Pine Tops Rd.**, named for the towering trees that shade its course, forms a 1.9-mile loop. Starting to the right of the building and following the loop in the counter-clockwise direction, the road heads north with a series of gentle slopes and curves amidst huge tree trunks and outcroppings of ledge. It reaches a high point after a third of a mile and descends past **Pine Tops Picnic Area**, then turns west and climbs to **Pearce Lake** after 0.8 miles where toilets (in summer) and a beautiful beach offer a spot to rest.

Pine Tops Rd. loops back to the visitor center with much hillier conditions. It climbs above the lake on several steep slopes which are followed by curving descents, then passes another picnic area and a view over **Silver Lake** at the 1.5-mile mark. Most of the remaining 0.4 miles back to the trailhead are downhill.

The reservation's longest loop combines Pine Tops Rd.

with two other roads for a 2.8-mile ride. **Elm Rd.** intersects at Pearce Lake's beach and runs for a half-mile, meandering through woods and gentle terrain to a set of powerlines at the trailhead near **Wakefield High School** and a **vocational school**.

Hemlock Rd. intersects on the left at this point and returns to the visitor center with a 1.3-mile rollercoaster of hills through the reservation's most challenging terrain. Guardrails along the shoulders lend a sense of security at several precipitous drops. Hemlock Rd. reaches a high point above Pearce Lake after a half-mile, drops steeply for the next quarter-mile to the water level, then combines strenuous ups and downs for the last half-mile back to Pine Tops Rd. Bear right at the end to reach the visitor center.

BACKGROUND:

Breakheart earned its name during the Civil War when troops utilized the area as a training ground and found it heartbreaking to be stationed at the remote and lonely site. Its 600 acres became public property in 1934 and served as a camp for the Civilian Conservation Corps during the Great Depression when roads, trails, and picnic areas were constructed. The state's Dept. of Conservation & Recreation manages the property.

DRIVING DIRECTIONS:

• **Visitor Center (Saugus):** From I-95/Rte. 128 take Exit 44 and follow Rte. 1 south for 2.5 miles. Exit at signs for Lynn Fells Pkwy. west, continue for a third of a mile, then turn right on Forest St. and park at the end.

• **Hemlock Rd. (Wakefield):** From I-95/Rte. 128, take Exit 44 and follow Rte. 1 south for 2 miles. Exit at signs for Rte. 129 west and drive for 2 miles, turn left on Farm Rd., then left on Hemlock Rd. Park at the trailhead at the end.

TOILETS:

visitor center, Pearce Lake (during swimming season)

ADDITIONAL INFORMATION:

Breakheart Reservation, (781) 233-0834
Dept. of Conservation & Recreation, mass.gov/dcr

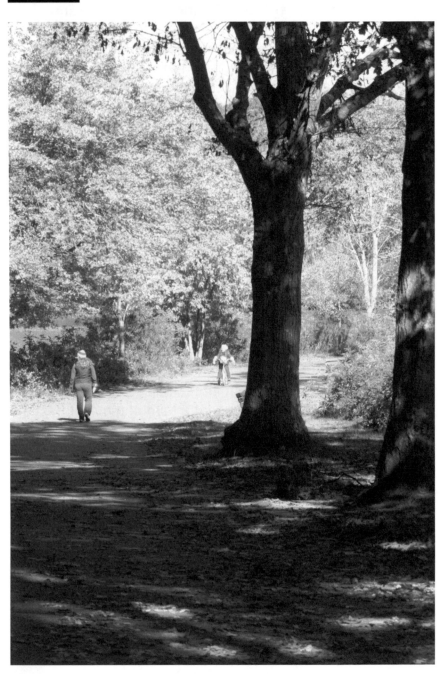

LENGTH: 8.8 miles including sections of on-road bike route
SURFACE: paved, plus some gravel trails at Horn Pond
TERRAIN: small slopes (except for Horn Pond Mtn.)

This combination of separated paths and on-road bike routes threads a welcoming course through an array of surroundings, joining 3 town centers with a quiet alternative.

RULES & SAFETY:
- Bicyclists should yield to pedestrians.
- Keep to the right, pass on the left, and alert others (*"On your left..."*) when approaching from behind.
- Several road crossings deserve extra caution. Stop at intersections and remember that drivers might not see you.
- *Bike Route* sections are open to car traffic.
- Horn Pond is a water supply so strict rules apply.
- Pets must be leashed and their wastes removed.

ORIENTATION:
The most car-free riding and natural scenery await at Woburn's Horn Pond. Road crossings are frequent near Winchester and Stoneham centers and several involve high-traffic areas that deserve extra caution. The separated path is interrupted by several on-road sections which are labeled with *Bike Route* markings. Terrain is flat in the area of the MBTA Commuter Rail but sloped on the approach to Stoneham center and in the surroundings of Horn Pond.

TRAIL DESCRIPTION:
Begin at **Horn Pond Recreation Area** in Woburn where a 2.1-mile loop circles a beautiful water view. From the **Lake Ave.** trailhead, follow the pathway uphill behind the water treatment facility and turn right on Cove St., a gated road. Fork right and continue north on **Woburn Pkwy.** past Lions Park (0.6 miles) and across a causeway separating "the lagoon," then keep right along the northern shore (1.1 miles) past a boat launch. Continue uphill and turn south on a gravel trail to Lynch Park (1.5 miles), then follow sidewalks beside **Arlington Rd.** and Lake Ave. to return to the trailhead. Unpaved trails branch westward at the lagoon into

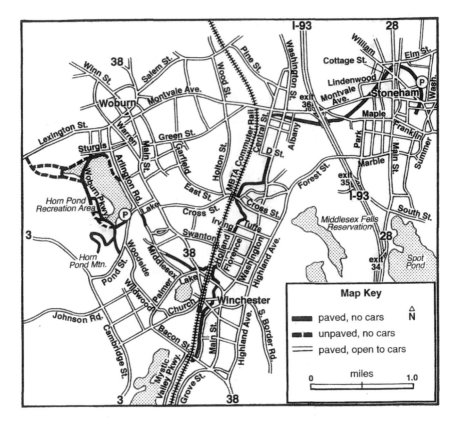

more natural scenery with narrower but generally smooth
gravel surfaces, while a strenuous ride climbs in switchbacks
from Woburn Pkwy. to the summit of 287' **Horn Pond Mtn.**
for a view over the Boston area.

To ride the Tri-Community Greenway, turn left on Lake
Ave. then immediately right on Lake Terrace and follow the
paved trail at the end of the street into Winchester along the
former Middlesex Canal. Continue straight on Sylvester Ave.
and **Middlesex St.**, fork left on Horn Pond Brook Rd. to the
Horn Pond Bikeway, then turn left beside **Lake St.** (1.0 mile).
After crossing **Main St./Rte. 38**, the trail skirts a ball field and
passes under **MBTA Commuter Rail** tracks to reach a T-
intersection beside Winchester High School (1.3 miles).

Turning right (south), the greenway extends for 1 mile
to **Bacon St.** following a slender space along the Aberjona
River through downtown **Winchester** where bicyclists are

144

advised to dismount at several intersections in order to use sidewalks that connect nearby crosswalks.

Turning left (north), the greenway extends for 3.8 miles to **Stoneham**. This leg soon turns right on Spruce St., left on **Holland**, right on **Swanton**, left on **Florence**, and left on **Irving**. The trail resumes on the right heading north past the Muraco School, along the Aberjona River, and across **Cross St.** before emerging at **Washington St.** (2.3 miles from Horn Pond). Here it turns left on a wide sidewalk for a quarter-mile, crosses the Woburn line, and follows *Bike Route* signs along **D St.** and **Central St.** through an area of cemeteries. The final leg is a rail-trail branching eastward on the right, crossing Washington St. and the Aberjona, passing under **I-93** at the Stoneham line, and climbing a noticeable slope to a cluster of road intersections including busy **Montvale Ave.**, **Main St./Rte. 28**, and Central St. The trail circles southward past a school and small trailhead before ending at Gould St., 5.1 miles from the Horn Pond trailhead.

BACKGROUND:

The Tri-Community Greenway opened in 2018 after a 30-year effort. It utilizes a former railroad at the Stoneham end, local greenspaces along the Aberjona River, and a reconstructed Horn Pond Bikeway. To the south, proposed trail construction along the Mystic Lakes would connect the Alewife Brook Greenway (Chap. 40).

Horn Pond has been designated common land since Woburn originated in 1640. It became a resort in the early 1800's when the Middlesex Canal, a 27-mile water route between Boston and Lowell, operated along what is now Arlington St. and drew passengers to the pond's pristine shores. It also supported a large ice cutting industry through the 1800's and became a water supply in 1873 using a reservoir on top of nearby Horn Pond Mtn.

DRIVING DIRECTIONS:

From I-95/Rte. 128: Take Exit 35 and follow Rte. 38 south for 2.3 miles. Turn right on Lake Ave. just before the Winchester town line and continue for a third of a mile. Look for the trailhead parking on the right beside the pond.

TOILETS:

Horn Pond trailhead

ADDITIONAL INFORMATION:

Tri-Community Greenway, tricommunitygreenway.org

Battle Road Trail
Lexington-Concord

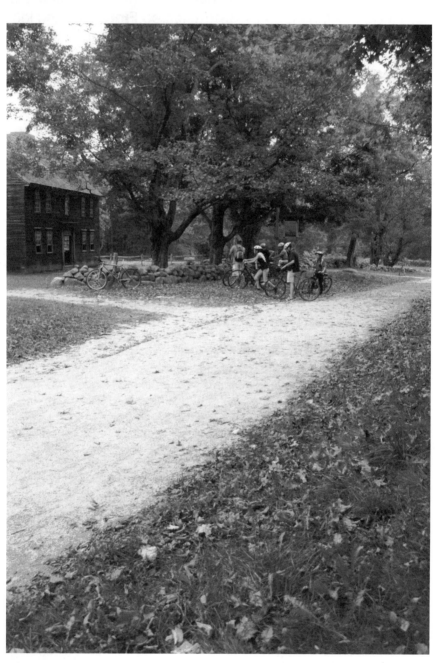

LENGTH: 4.8 miles
SURFACE: stone dust
TERRAIN: moderate slopes
NOTE: wide-tired bicycles preferable

A passage through time, the Minute Man National Historic Park's trail blends recreation, nature, and history like no other bike path in the state.

RULES & SAFETY:

- Bicyclists should yield to pedestrians.
- Keep to the right, pass on the left, and alert others (*"On your left..."*) when approaching from behind.
- The trail is designed for slow-speed bicycling and is relatively narrow and curvy in places.
- Bicyclists are requested to walk at boardwalks.
- Stay on the trail and be sensitive to the private property, farmland, and archeological sites surrounding it.
- Dogs must be leashed and their wastes removed.
- Parking lots close each day at sunset.

ORIENTATION:

The Battle Road Tr. parallels Rte. 2A in the east-west direction and, for much of the way, follows a historic route used in the battle of April 19, 1775. Sections of original "Battle Road" and most of the historic sites lie along the eastern two thirds of the trail while farmland and forest predominate at the western end. Three major trailheads are shown on the map while additional parking lots also exist. Historic sites are marked by interpretive signs beside the trail and, together with a few intersecting roads, provide helpful points of reference. Note that Hanscom Field, located just north of the trail, is a source of low-flying aircraft.

TRAIL DESCRIPTION:

Start at the Visitor Ctr. trailhead in Lincoln and follow the connecting trail from the parking lot to the Battle Road, which is lined by stone walls. Turning right (east), a mile of trail extends into Lexington to **I-95/Rte. 128**, first crossing **Airport Rd.** and paralleling **Marrett St./Rte. 2A** in flat terrain

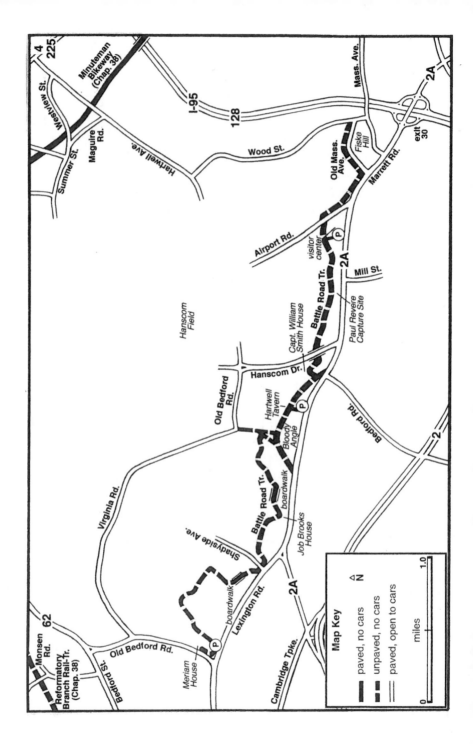

and then arcing left and following **Old Mass. Ave.** up a long slope on **Fiske Hill** and descending to **Wood St.**

Heading west from the Visitor Ctr., the trail extends for 3.8 miles. The trip begins beside stone walls of the original Battle Road then detours at the **Paul Revere Capture Site**, passes through a tunnel under **Hanscom Dr.** (0.8 miles), and curves past the **Capt. William Smith House.** Turning right on another segment of the old road, the trail rises on a gradual slope to **Hartwell Tavern** (1.4 miles) where park employees occasionally await in period dress and offer tours of the building. Parking and toilets are located nearby.

The Battle Road Tr. continues west to an intersection at **Bloody Angle** (1.6 miles) and turns right. Leaving the old road, it runs north briefly and then turns left at a sign, descending through woods to a boardwalk at a wetland. The trail enters Concord on the other side and climbs past the **Job Brooks House**, emerges at **Lexington Rd.** and **Shadyside Ave.** (2.6 miles), and returns to woods with a downhill slope to a second boardwalk. It traces farm fields before reaching the western trailhead (3.6 miles) on Lexington Rd. and ends at the **Miriam House** on **Old Bedford Rd.** (3.8 miles).

BACKGROUND:

Minute Man National Historic Park preserves the Battle of April 19, 1775, the start of the American Revolutionary War. It occupies the route between Lexington and Concord that British troops followed in a failed attempt to capture munitions and quell unrest.

Construction of the Battle Road Tr. began in 1997 and incorporated a unique sand/clay surface which met the needs for universal accessibility as well as a historical and natural appearance.

DRIVING DIRECTIONS:

From I-95/Rte. 128: Take Exit 30B and follow Rte. 2A west for 1 mile to the Visitor Center entrance on the right.

For Hartwell Tavern, continue on Rte. 2A west for one additional mile and look for the parking lot on the right.

TOILETS:

Visitor Ctr., Hartwell Tavern, Miriam House

ADDITIONAL INFORMATION:

Minute Man Nat'l Historic Park, (978)369-6993, www.nps.gov/mima

38 Minuteman Bikeway
Bedford-Cambridge

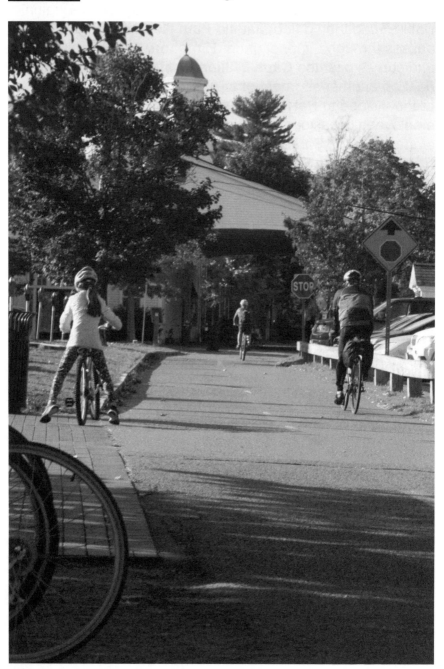

LENGTH: 10.1 miles, plus side trails
SURFACE: paved
TERRAIN: slight slopes

The state's most popular rail-trail stays in motion throughout the year connecting the city and the suburbs with a steady stream of commuting, exercise, and family fun. High levels of use require especially cautious trail manners.

RULES & SAFETY:
- Bicyclists should yield to pedestrians.
- Keep to the right, pass on the left, and alert others (*"On your left..."*) when approaching from behind.
- Be especially cautious in the presence of children and pets since their movements can be unpredictable.
- Groups should ride single file.
- Step off the trail when stopped so others can pass.
- Stop at road intersections and remember that drivers might not be aware of your presence.
- Respect nearby residents by keeping noise levels low.
- Pets must be leashed and their wastes removed.
- Horses and motorized vehicles are prohibited.
- Watch for additional information posted at trailheads.

ORIENTATION:
Several trailheads provide a choice of starting points and are easiest to find along the northwestern portion of the bikeway. Visitors should note that the Thorndike Field parking lot near the trail's southeast end has a two-hour limit and serves playing fields which can be crowded.

Natural scenery is best along a 4-mile segment of trail between the centers of Lexington and Arlington, and this section also benefits from a lack of road intersections. The trail has a noteworthy detour from the original rail line at a busy downtown intersection in Arlington center which requires either walking along sidewalks or riding with car traffic. Elevation changes along the route are minimal but slight slopes reach a high point at Lexington center.

The Minuteman Bikeway connects several other trails:

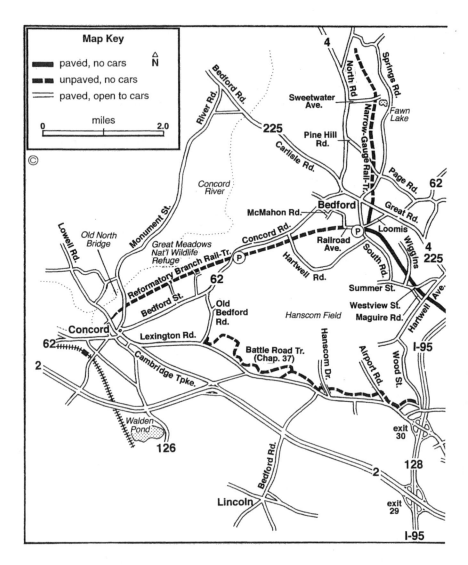

the unpaved, 2.9-mile Narrow Gauge Rail-Trail heads north from Bedford to the Billerica town line; the unpaved, 3.9-mile Reformatory Branch Rail-Trail heads west from Bedford to Concord center, and the Alewife area bike paths (Chap. 40) extend from the southeast endpoint in Cambridge at the Alewife T Station. Nearby, the parallel Battle Road Tr. (Chapter 37) does not intersect but runs between Lexington and Concord.

TRAIL DESCRIPTION:

Starting in **Bedford**, the bikeway heads southeast from the Depot Park trailhead on **South Rd.** beside a restored train car and visitor center. It straightens along a woodsy corridor to the crossing of **Wiggins Ave.** (1.0 mile) near the Shawsheen River and the Lexington town line, intersects **Westview St.** (1.2 miles), and then reaches busy **Hartwell Ave.** (1.4 miles) at a traffic signal. A slight uphill

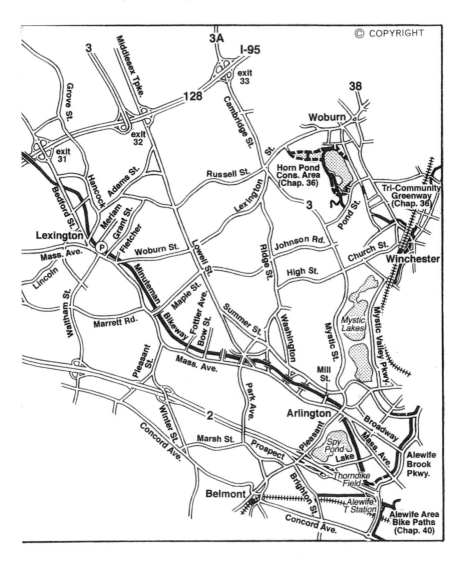

© COPYRIGHT

slope affects the next two miles as the bikeway passes over 8-lane **I-95/Rte. 128** (2.0 miles) and intersects **Bedford St./Rte. 4/225** (2.6 miles) at another signaled crosswalk.

Flattening at the crossing of **Hancock St.** (3.7 miles), it meets a cluster of intersections in **Lexington** center and passes the historic town green, site of the first shots of the Revolutionary War. Just ahead, the trail slips through an original covered train station beside a public parking lot.

A slight downslope carries the trail for most of the next 4.5 miles. After crossing **Woburn St.** (4.3 miles), it enters the natural scenery of conservation lands and intersects fewer roads, passing underneath **Maple St.** (5.3 miles) along this stretch. The trail crosses **Bow St.** (6.3 miles) and then enters Arlington where homes and businesses line both sides but bridges allow it to pass either over or under roads for the next 2 miles to **Mill St.** (8.3 miles).

The trail is disrupted at **Mystic St.** (8.6 miles) in downtown **Arlington** where a short detour is required by either walking on sidewalks or carefully riding along busy streets. Turn right on Mystic, turn left on **Mass. Ave.** while crossing to its south side, and then turn right on Swan Place to rejoin the rail-trail (8.7 miles) on the left side.

The remaining distance travels through residential neighborhoods in leafy surroundings. The trail gets a view of **Spy Pond** on the right before **Lake St.** (9.5 miles), emerges at **Thorndike Field** (9.8 miles), and intersects Alewife Brook Greenway (Chap. 38) on the left before passing underneath **Rte. 2** (9.9 miles) in Cambridge. The bikeway ends at the **Alewife T Station** (10.1 miles), a hub for other bike paths in the area (Chap. 38).

Extending from the Bedford end, the 2.9-mile **Narrow-Gauge Rail-Trail** has easy biking and woodsy surroundings. From the end of the bikeway, turn right on South Rd. and immediately right on **Loomis St.**, then watch for the trail on the left at a gate. Asphalt covers the first third of a mile to **Great Rd./Rte. 4/225** and a stone dust surface continues past conservation lands to **Sweetwater Ave.** (2.0 miles) near

Fawn Lake and the Billerica town line (2.9 miles).

The 4.0-mile **Reformatory Branch Rail-Trail** joins Bedford and Concord centers with a mostly smooth, dirt surface which will be upgraded along the Bedford portion. From the bikeway, turn right on South Rd., immediately left on **Railroad Ave.**, and find the trail a third of a mile straight ahead at a sharp right turn. It intersects **Hartwell Rd.** (0.9 miles) and **Rte. 62** (1.7 miles) before entering Concord, passes the **Great Meadows Wildlife Refuge**, then contends with a bumpier surface on the way to **Monument St.** (3.7 miles) near Minuteman Nat'l. Park's Old North Bridge. A narrower path continues to **Lowell Rd.** (4.0 miles).

BACKGROUND:

The Minuteman Bikeway follows the route of a railroad which was built from North Cambridge to Lexington in 1846 and extended to Bedford in 1874. The last train ran in 1981, trail construction began in 1991, and the Minuteman opened as the country's 500th rail-trail in 1993. Later inducted in the Rails-to-Trails Conservancy's Hall of Fame, it ranks among the country's most popular.

The adjoining Narrow-Gauge Rail-Trail follows the former Billerica & Bedford Railroad which was completed in 1877 as the country's first two-foot-gauge, common-carrier railway. The Reformatory Branch, built in 1879, facilitated construction of the Concord Reformatory but missing bridges over the Sudbury and Assabet rivers now limit the trail to Lowell Rd. in Concord. The Bedford portion of this trail will soon be improved beyond Rte. 62.

DRIVING DIRECTIONS:

• **Depot Park, Bedford trailhead:** From I-95/Rte. 128 take Exit 31B and follow Rte. 4 north/Rte. 225 west for 1.9 miles. Turn left on Loomis St., continue straight at the next 4-way intersection, and park in the lot behind the bike shop immediately on the left.

• **Lexington center trailhead:** From I-95/Rte. 128 take Exit 31A and follow Rte. 4 south/Rte. 225 east for 1.7 miles. Turn left after Meriam St. at Depot Sq. and park in the municipal lot straight ahead.

TOILETS:

Depot Park (Bedford), Lexington visitor center, Alewife T station

ADDITIONAL INFORMATION:

minutemanbikeway.org

39 Wayside Rail-Trail
Wayland-Weston

LENGTH: 4.9 miles
SURFACE: mostly paved, some stone dust
TERRAIN: mostly flat, some small slopes

This long-awaited section of the Mass. Central passes lots of quiet conservation land as it joins two town centers.
RULES & SAFETY:
- Bicyclists should yield to pedestrians.
- Keep to the right, pass on the left, and alert others *"On your left..."*) when approaching from behind.
- Dogs should have short leashes and wastes removed.
- The trail is open from dawn until dusk.
- Areas of trail under construction are closed to use.

ORIENTATION:
Trailheads provide access in each town, and road crossings have crosswalks and signs. Elevation changes are minimal but a high point exists near Conant Rd. and low points exist at each end. The trail follows the treeless corridor of a powerline so it is fully exposed to the sun.

The rail-trail is currently divided in two parts by Conant Rd. where the site of a former bridge over the railroad has been filled, blocking the trail. Future construction will provide a tunnel through the embankment to join both sides.

TRAIL DESCRIPTION:
Begin at the west end where the **Wayland Town Ctr.** commercial area provides parking off **Rte. 20**. The trail's stone dust surface leads eastward beside the parking lot following a utility corridor and soon reaches **Wayland Depot** at the signaled crosswalk for **Rte. 27/126** (0.5 miles). The surface changes to asphalt and straightens with the utility poles along a 2.5-mile line rippled with small ups and downs. After crossing **Plain Rd.** (1.8 miles), it enters Weston where much of the surrounding woods are protected conservation

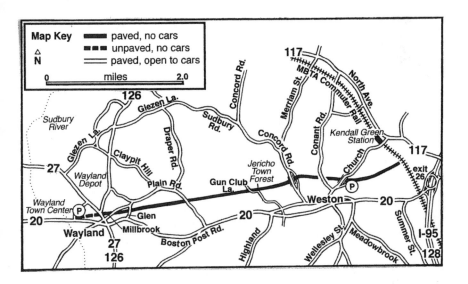

lands including **Jericho Town Forest**, which is accessed just past private **Gun Club La.** (2.7 miles). The trail passes under **Concord Rd.** (3.3 miles) and then gets blocked by an embankment at **Conant Rd.** (3.7 miles) where future tunnel construction will connect the next leg. A footpath currently climbs this slope to the road and descends the other side. Continuing, the rail-trail passes under **Church St.** (4.0 miles) at a trailhead and former station, then ends before a bridge over the **MBTA Fitchburg Commuter Rail Line** (4.9 miles).

BACKGROUND:

This route originated as the Massachusetts Central Railroad, built between Boston and Northampton in 1887 and operated until 1938 when a hurricane ended through service. Owned by the MBTA, the Waltham-Berlin portion was leased in 2011 to the state's Dept. of Conservation & Recreation which built this section of trail in a cooperative effort with Eversource, a utility company in need of a service road for powerlines. Extensions are planned at both ends.

DRIVING DIRECTIONS:

From I-95, take Exit 26 and follow signs off the rotary for Rte. 20 west. After 5.2 miles, and a half-mile beyond the intersection of Rte. 27/126, turn right at "Wayland Town Ctr." and park at the south end of the lot beside the powerlines.

ADDITIONAL INFORMATION:

masscentralrailtrail.org

40 Alewife Area Bike Paths

Cambridge, Arlington, Somerville

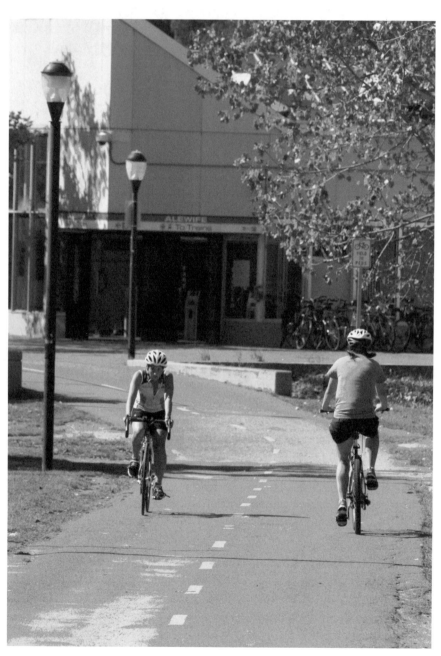

LENGTH: 10 miles
SURFACE: mostly paved, some stone dust
TERRAIN: mostly flat with a few small slopes

A growing, and glowing, network of bike paths helps make Alewife both a well-used hub for car-free travel and an accessible resource for recreation.

RULES & SAFETY:
- Bicyclists should yeild to pedestrians.
- Keep to the right, pass on the left, and alert others (*"On your left..."*) when approaching from behind.
- Be extra cautious when children or pets are present.
- Dogs must be leashed and their wastes removed.
- Swimming, wading, and other acts that degrade the water quality at Fresh Pond are prohibited.
- Note that some of the area's trailhead parking lots are restricted by either time limits, resident permit requirements, or capacity during athletic events.

ORIENTATION:
Bike paths extend in all directions with a variety of conditions. The flattest choices follow rail-trails and Alewife Brook for out-and-back rides but encounter frequent road intersections. Alternatively, several parks offer loops through somewhat hillier terrain with fewer road crossings.

TRAIL DESCRIPTIONS:
Begin at Cambridge's **Mayor Danehy Park** where 2 miles of paved trails circle ball fields, a playground, and picnic tables in a landscaped, hilltop setting. A wide, central trail leads from the **New St.** parking lot over a gradual slope to another lot on **Sherman St.** near the park headquarters. Other trails branch from this including a left-hand option at the midpoint which heads uphill for a view over the park.

Mild terrain surrounding nearby **Fresh Pond** creates a popular, 2.3-mile loop accessible by signaled crosswalks on **Fresh Pond Pkwy.** Note that walkers use this trail in great numbers so cyclists should ride cautiously. Circling in the clockwise direction, the trail parallels the parkway for a

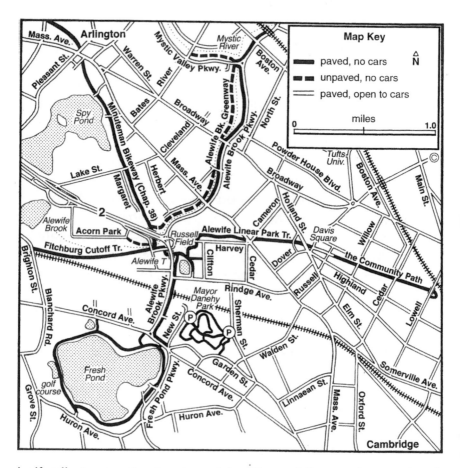

half-mile to a water treatment facility and then enjoys natural surroundings past a **golf course** and Little Fresh Pond.

The 2-mile **Alewife Linear Park Tr.** heads east from Alewife T Station. The paved path passes under **Alewife Brook Pkwy.**, turns left at **Russell Field**, crosses **Harvey St.**, and joins the route of the former Mass. Central R.R. It negotiates 3 crosswalks at **Mass. Ave.** (0.7 miles), then enters Somerville where it's known as **the Community Path**. Just ahead, **Davis Square** (1.1 miles) disrupts the route with a T station, pedestrian plaza, and road intersections which deserve caution, but an imaginary straight line leads to the next section of trail at the end of a parking lot beyond Grove St. The path intersects **Willow Ave.** (1.5 miles) and **Cedar St.** (1.8 miles) before ending at **Lowell St.** (2.0 miles).

Heading in the opposite direction, the 0.8-mile **Fitchburg Cutoff Tr.** follows the same line west into Belmont. It begins at the Alewife T Station, passes office buildings on Cambridge Park Dr. and walking trails along **Alewife Brook**, merges beside the Fitchburg Commuter Rail Line, and ends at **Brighton St.** (0.8 miles).

The 10-mile **Minuteman Bikeway** (Chap. 38) leaves from the same point at Alewife heading north under Concord Tpke./**Rte. 2** to Arlington, Lexington, and Bedford. The 1.8-mile **Alewife Brook Greenway Bike Path** intersects on the right as the Minuteman exits the Rte. 2 underpass and follows the greenspace of Alewife Brook downstream to the **Mystic River**. The path utilizes boardwalks at low areas and signaled crosswalks at busy intersections with **Mass. Ave.** (0.5 miles), **Broadway** (1.0 mile), **Mystic Valley Pkwy.** (1.5 miles), and **Boston Ave.** (1.8 miles). Trail segments on the Arlington side of the brook have a smooth, stone dust surface and surprisingly natural surroundings while those on the Cambridge and Somerville side are paved and follow busy Alewife Brook Pkwy. A quarter-mile-long trail with a stone dust surface intersects near the end and extends westward along the Mystic River.

BACKGROUND:

Built over many years, these bike paths have a variety of origins. Mayor Danehy Park was created in 1991 on the site of a former city landfill. Fresh Pond, Cambridge's water supply since 1852, and its perimeter trail have long been a popular greenspace and will be joined to Watertown and the Charles River Reservation (Chap. 45) by future construction of a rail-trail. Alewife Linear Park was established in the 1980's with the construction of the Red Line subway to Alewife, and the Community Path extended this route in 1995. The Alewife Brook Greenway Bike Path was completed in 2012 and will link a future trail planned along the Mystic River.

DRIVING DIRECTIONS:

Mayor Danehy Park: Follow Rte. 2 east along Alewife Brook Pkwy. to Fresh Pond Pkwy. At Brodette Circle, turn left on New St. and find the park on the right after 0.3 miles.

TOILETS:

Mayor Danehy Park, Alewife T Station, Fresh Pond

Mystic River Reservation
Medford & Somerville

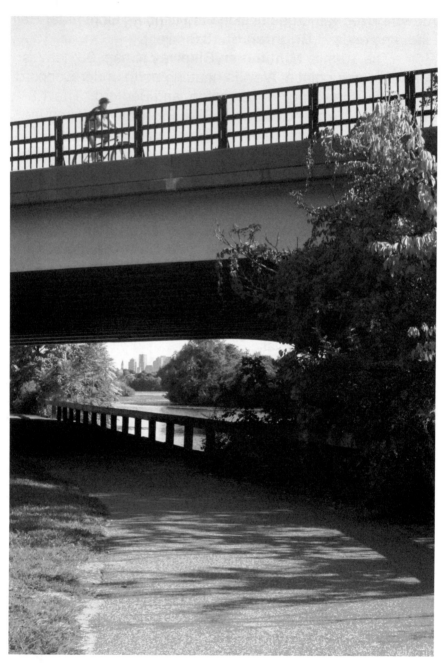

LENGTH: 4.8 miles
SURFACE: paved
TERRAIN: small slopes

This cluster of trails at the outskirts of the city connects neighboring parks on both sides of the Mystic River and will be a future crossroad of regional bike paths.

RULES & SAFETY:
- Bicyclists should yield to pedestrians.
- Keep to the right, pass on the left, and alert others (*"On your left..."*) when approaching from behind.
- Be extra cautious when children and pets are present since their movements can be unpredictable.
- Step off the trail when stopped so others can pass.
- Pets must be leashed and their wastes removed.
- The reservation is open only during daylight hours.

ORIENTATION:
The centerpiece of the reservation is MacDonald Park, an area of lawns, benches, and shade trees beside the Mystic River. Paved trails extend in all directions and utilize bridges and underpasses to link surrounding greenspaces while avoiding road intersections. Use of sidewalks is required at a few points. Trails are not marked but the riverbank location is a helpful point of reference for first-time visitors. The area's bike paths range in age with older ones having relatively narrow width and inferior surfaces and the newer ones being generally wider and smoother.

TRAIL DESCRIPTION:
Beginning at the trailhead parking lot on **Mystic Valley Pkwy./Rte. 16**, head west through **MacDonald Park's** network of paved loops which explore enjoyable scenery along the **Mystic River**. A perimeter route through this area measures 0.9 miles from the trailhead. Watch for a 3-story observation **tower** offering an excellent view over the river to the skyline of Boston. Just beyond this, the trail splits at Rte. 16's **Veterans Memorial Bridge** with a sidewalk leading across the river and an underpass allowing

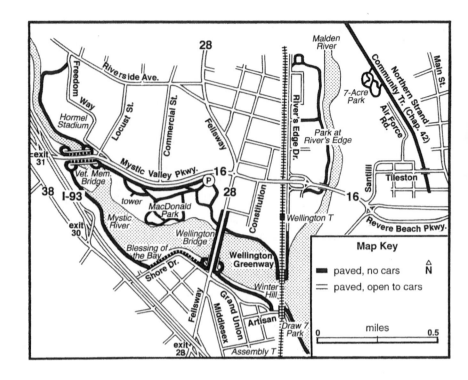

the trail to slip beneath the road.

Fork left and descend under the bridge to access another mile of bike paths north of the parkway. Athletic facilities at **Hormel Stadium** attract most of the attention in this area while a paved trail explores the riverbank with smooth rolling in a quiet, landscaped setting.

For a longer ride venture to the opposite side of the Mystic where a 2-mile stretch of trail awaits. Cross Veterans Memorial Bridge using the sidewalks on either side of the road and the bike path underpasses on either side of the river. Heading south (left) on the other side, the path follows a narrow strip of land between the river and **I-93** offering views over the water but also plenty of highway noise for part of the way. After entering Somerville, it reaches **Blessing of the Bay Boat House** (1.4 miles from the trailhead parking lot), where benches look across to the reservation's grassy slopes, and then joins a sidewalk at the edge of **Shore Dr.** for a third of a mile.

Approaching **Fellsway/Rte. 28**, the trail curves left and utilizes a boardwalk built over the water to pass under the **Wellington Bridge**. Bending back on the other side, the paved pathway continues downstream through landscaped waterfront parkland alongside the Assembly Square Mall and the **Winter Hill Yacht Club**, passes under a commuter rail line near the dam and locks which contain the river, and ends at **Draw Seven Park**.

The Wellington Bridge allows safe bike/pedestrian passage across the river along both sides of Rte. 28. Returning to Medford on the north side, turn left (west) to reach the trailhead or turn right (east) along the riverbank to ride the **Wellington Greenway**, a bike path which wraps underneath a railroad bridge and turns north to link **Wellington T Station**. Another mile of pathway extends northward under Rte. 16 and upstream along the **Malden River** through **the Park at River's Edge**. Future trail construction will connect the nearby **Northern Strand Community Tr.** (Chap. 42).

BACKGROUND:

The Mystic River Reservation originated in the 1960's when construction of I-93 eliminated three large bends in the river and filled acres of wetland. Since that time, parkland has been refurbished and expanded in conjunction with nearby bridge construction and waterfront development projects.

The reservation lies at the crossroads of surrounding bike paths and future trail construction is expected to link these routes. Connections are planned with the Alewife Brook Greenway (Chapter 40), Northern Strand Community Tr. (Chapter 42), and the Charles River Reservation (Chapter 45).

DRIVING DIRECTIONS:

- **I-93 northbound:** Take Exit 29 and follow Rte. 28 north for 0.7 miles, turn left on Rte. 16 west, then immediately left at the trailhead parking lot.
- **I-93 southbound:** Take Exit 31, follow Rte. 16 east, and look for the parking lot less than a mile ahead on the right, just before Rte. 28.

ADDITIONAL INFORMATION:

Dept. of Conservation & Recreation, www.mass.gov/dcr

Northern Strand Community Tr.

Everett-Lynn

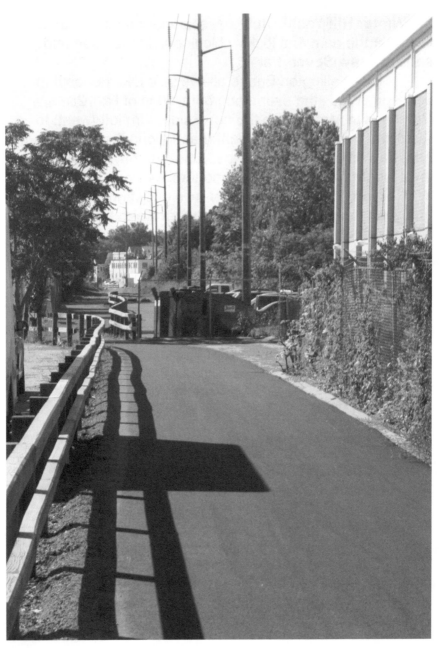

LENGTH: 7.6 miles
SURFACE: half is paved, half is processed stone/gravel
TERRAIN: flat
NOTE: wide-tired bikes recommended for unpaved sections

A local effort known as *Bike to the Sea* reclaimed this former rail line as a valuable refuge for cyclists and walkers.

RULES & SAFETY:
- Bicyclists should yield to pedestrians.
- Keep to the right, pass on the left, and alert others (*"On your left..."*) when approaching from behind.
- Pets must be leashed and their wastes removed.
- The trail is open only during daylight hours.

ORIENTATION:
The 4-mile, paved southwestern portion in Malden and Everett has an urban setting and limited shade while the 3.6-mile, unpaved northeastern section in Revere and Saugus has a woodsy, residential environment and natural scenery. The trail offers crosswalks at road intersections and occasional benches and information kiosks. The undeveloped, 1.4-mile trail in Lynn is merely a footpath.

TRAIL DESCRIPTION:
Heading southwest (turning left when facing the trail) from the **Beach St.** trailhead, the paved bike path stretches for 4 miles. It begins along a corridor of utility poles for the first mile and a half, passing a variety of businesses and two schools while intersecting busy **Broadway/Rte. 99** (0.7 miles) and **Maplewood St.** (1.0 mile). The trail encounters a cluster of side streets and follows a narrower passageway on the approach to downtown **Malden** where it meets **Rte. 60** (2.1 miles), **Ferry St.** (2.2 miles), and **Main St.** (2.4 miles). Use extra caution at these major intersections.

Fencing corrals the trail through an industrial area as it departs downtown and turns south along Canal St. near the **Malden River.** After a final road crossing at **Medford St.** (2.9 miles), it enters Everett and continues past **7-Acre Park** where side trails join on the right. The last half-mile parallels

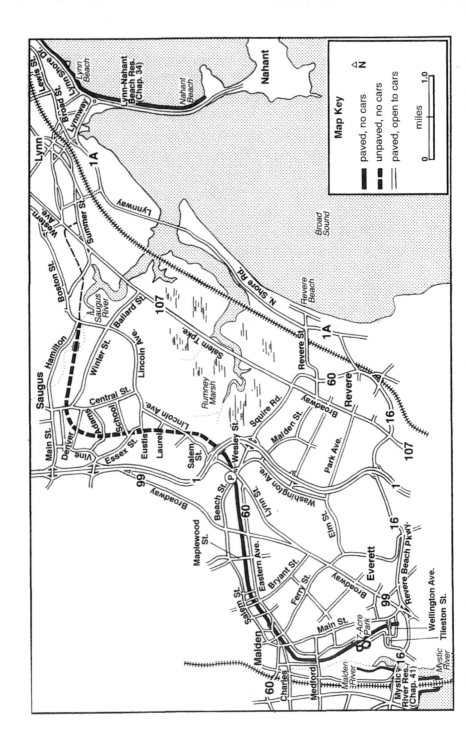

Air Force Rd., passes under **Tileston St.**, and currently ends at **Wellington Ave.** (4.0 miles) before a **Rte. 16** underpass.

Riding northeast from Beach St. in Malden, the Northern Strand extends for 3.6 miles. It crosses **Lynn St.** and Wesley St., enters Revere where the asphalt surface changes to a compacted material, and passes under **Rte. 1** (0.4 miles) with a view across **Rumney Marsh**. After curving northward to **Salem St.** (0.9 miles), the trail enters woods on an aggregate surface at the Saugus line near **Laurel St.** (1.2 miles), passes a former station house at **Eustis St.**, and emerges beside Anna Parker Playground. It continues across the intersection of **Essex St.** and **School St.** (1.6 miles), crosses **Adams St.** (2.0 miles), and makes a long, eastward curve past two schools and **Denver St.** (2.3 miles).

The trail cuts through a small parking lot before crossing **Central St.** (2.6 miles) near downtown **Saugus** and straightens, heading east and eventually emerging in open marshland along the **Saugus River**. Old asphalt smoothens the surface and a bridge over the river (3.4 miles) allows a broad view before the trail ends at **Lincoln Ave.** (3.6 miles) and the Lynn city line. A footpath continues eastward from this point beside the old railroad tracks for another 1.4 miles to **Summer St.** but has not been developed for bicycling.

BACKGROUND:

This route originated in 1853 as the Saugus Branch Railroad and eventually connected Boston and Lynn. When train service ended, the volunteer group *Bike to the Sea* formed in 1993 to promote the creation of a rail-trail and the first sections opened in 2012 and 2013. The Northern Strand Community Tr. is envisioned to reach north to the beaches of Lynn (Chapter 34) and Revere and south to the Mystic River Reservation (Chapter 41). It is a designated part of the E. Coast Greenway, a route being developed from Maine to Florida.

DRIVING DIRECTIONS:

Beach St., Malden: From Rte. 1, exit at Rte. 60 and drive west toward Malden for 0.3 miles. Where Rte. 60 turns left at Lynn St., continue straight on Beach St. and park in the lot immediately on the right, or find street parking nearby.

ADDITIONAL INFORMATION:

biketothesea.com

43 Deer Island Park
Winthrop

LENGTH: 3.7 miles
SURFACE: paved
TERRAIN: flat perimeter loop, hilly side trails

This spectacular Boston Harbor location holds wide open scenery and cool summer breezes, but parking is scarce on popular days and wind can be a deterent on others.

RULES & SAFETY:
- Bicyclists should yield to pedestrians.
- Keep to the right, pass on the left, and alert others (*"On your left..."*) when approaching from behind.
- Do not block the trail when stopped.
- No rollerblading, skateboarding, or swimming.
- Dogs must be leashed and their wastes removed.
- The park is vulnerable to wind and adverse weather.
- The trail is open from sunrise to sunset.

ORIENTATION:
A flat, 2.7-mile perimeter loop follows the shoreline while side trails branch to interior hilltops with significant slopes and great views. The trails offer plenty of benches as well as interpretive signs about the area's history.

TRAIL DESCRIPTION:
Following the 2.7-mile **Deer Island Loop Tr.** in the clockwise direction from the parking lot, the trail rounds a slope to an easterly view of the Atlantic and follows a row of granite blocks along the peninsula's curving north shore. It then turns south on a seawall past the **sewage treatment facility** to the end of the peninsula (1.4 miles) where a grand view of the harbor, islands, and city skyline awaits.

Returning northward on the western side, the trail intersects access roads at **Gate 14** (1.6 miles) and **Gate 16** (1.8 miles), passes the **Main Entrance Gate**, and turns through natural surroundings along **Tafts Ave.** back to the

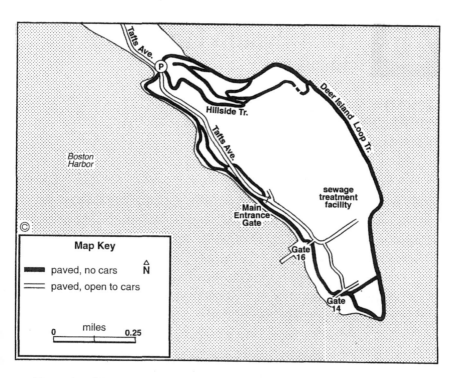

trailhead. Climb **Hillside Tr.** for the park's best view but use
caution when descending the slope.

BACKGROUND:

Named in the 1600's for its population of deer taking refuge from
wolves, this property has served as a quarantine station for
immigrants, an asylum for the poor, a reformatory for delinquents, a
prison, and a military post. Deer Island now holds a massive
sewage treatment facility for Boston and 43 communities in the
metropolitan area, protecting the harbor as one of the cleanest in the
nation. Part of Boston Harbor Islands National Recreation Area,
Deer Island is managed by the Mass. Water Resources Authority.

DRIVING DIRECTIONS:

From I-90, continue east past Logan Airport, merge
onto Rte. 1A north, turn right on Rte. 145, and continue east
for 3.5 miles. Where Rte. 145 turns left on Veterans Rd.,
continue straight on Washington Ave. Turn right on Shirley
St. and drive for one mile, turn left on Eliot St., turn right on
Tafts Ave., and park in the lot a third of a mile ahead.

TOILET FACILITIES:

Portable toilets at two points along the perimeter loop

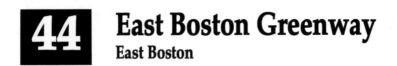

44 East Boston Greenway
East Boston

LENGTH: 2 miles, plus side trails
SURFACE: paved
TERRAIN: flat

Squeezing through a busy urban area, this landscaped greenway mingles with boats on the harbor, trains on the Blue Line, planes at Logan Airport, and the shadows of Rte. 1A bridges. Impressively, the path crosses only two streets.

RULES & SAFETY:
• Bicyclists should yield to pedestrians.
• Watch for separate, designated areas for pedestrians and bicyclists along some sections, otherwise keep right.
• Dogs are not welcome where the trail passes through Bremen Street Park, as posted by signs. In other areas, pets must be leashed and their wastes removed.

ORIENTATION:
Navigating the bike path's landscaped corridor is easy except at the crossing of Frankfort St. which can be confusing. Note that the northernmost 0.8 miles of the trail intersects no roads and is confined by fencing on both sides.

TRAIL DESCRIPTION:
Begin at **East Boston Mem. Park** where a mile of paved trails surround playing fields and a stadium. To the west, pass under Rte. 1A's bridges to reach East Boston Greenway (identified by its white center line) as it intersects other paved trails in neighboring **Bremen St. Park**.

Turning south (left), the greenway follows lamp poles and tree plantings along a below-ground corridor, passing under surrounding streets before ending near **Marginal St.** (0.5 miles) at a view of **Boston Inner Harbor** and the city.

Turning north (right), the greenway parallels Bremen St. Park's long area of lawns for the first half-mile past playgrounds, the Airport T Station, and the E. Boston Public

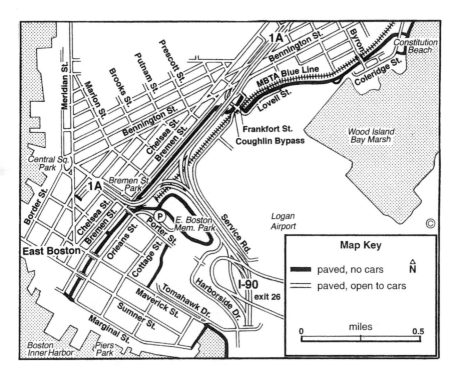

Library. The bike path continues under Rte. 1A (0.6 miles), intersects **Coughlin Bypass Rd.**, turns right and crosses **Frankfort St.**, and curves left between the MBTA Blue Line and **Lovell St.** With air traffic from **Logan Airport** overhead, the last stretch follows a fenced corridor past the Wood Island T Station and a view of **Wood Island Bay Marsh** before ending at **Constitution Beach** (1.5 miles).

BACKGROUND:

Following decades of hardship, East Boston's greenspace has been growing. This abandoned rail line, donated to the Boston Natural Areas Fund in 1996, has been transformed into a valuable greenway between neighborhoods, parks, and T stations. Future construction is planned to eventually bring the trail north to Belle Island Marsh Reservation.

DRIVING DIRECTIONS:

From I-93 in Boston, take Exit 24B for Rte. 1A north. After exiting the Callahan Tunnel take the "East Boston" exit and follow Porter St. for 3 blocks (with a "jog" left at Chelsea St.). Turn left on Orleans St. and park in the lot ahead.

Charles River Reservation
Boston-Newton

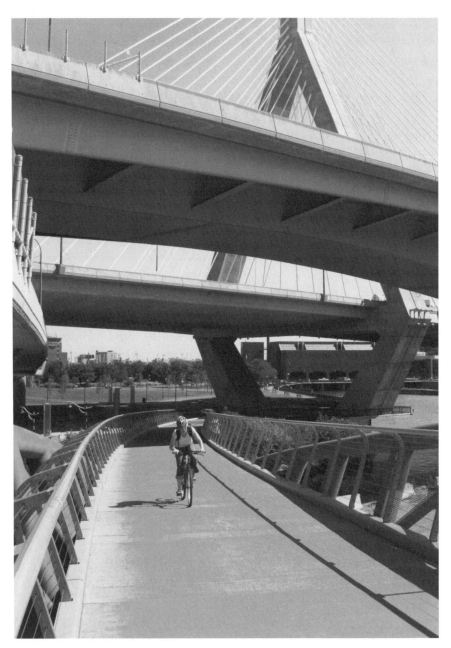

LENGTH: 25 miles
SURFACE: mostly paved
TERRAIN: small slopes

Convenient to millions, the state's most visible bike path follows a string of parks and natural areas along the river.

RULES & SAFETY:
- Bicyclists should yield to pedestrians.
- Keep to the right, pass on the left, and alert others (*"On your left..."*) when approaching from behind.
- Be extra cautious in crowded areas, and when children or pets are present since they can be unpredictable.
- Bicycling is not permitted on all of the reservation's trails. Watch for signs marking pedestrian-only trails.
- Wooden boardwalks are slippery when wet.
- Be cautious at road intersections since traffic can be busy and fast. Use crosswalks and signals where available.
- Dogs must be leashed and their wastes removed.

ORIENTATION:
Bike paths extend from landscaped, urban parks in Boston west to natural, woodsy areas in Newton. The Dr. Paul Dudley White Bike Path spans the eastern two thirds of this distance with paved trails along both banks of the river and bridge connections at numerous points. West of Watertown Sq., the Charles River Greenway is identified by a blue heron icon and forms a more disjointed course with a few gaps requiring on-road links.

TRAIL DESCRIPTION:
Beginning at the midsection at the **Soldiers Field Rd.** trailhead, the Dr. Paul Dudley White Bike Path makes a 10.7-mile loop in Cambridge and Boston. Facing the **Charles River**, turn right on the paved path, pass under the **Eliot Bridge**, keep right and cross the bridge over the river, then curve eastward along the north shore. The path follows **Memorial Dr.** for 5 miles, intersecting roads after a mile at Harvard University, joining a sidewalk at ramps for the B.U. Bridge (2.7 miles), straightening beside the river near M.I.T.,

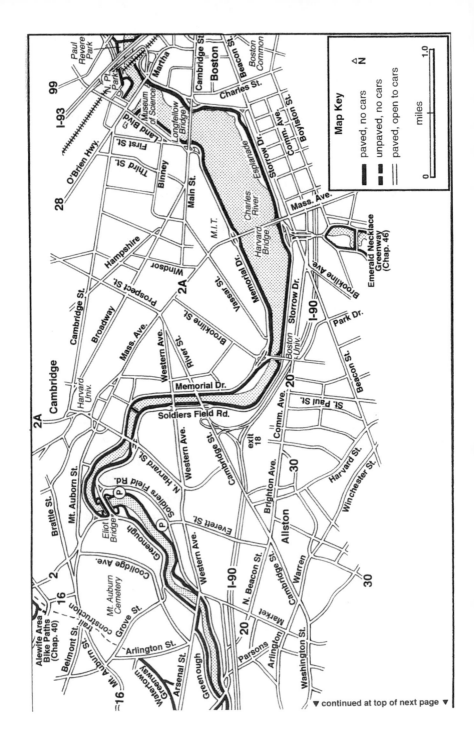

Map Key

paved, no cars	
unpaved, no cars	
paved, open to cars	

N

miles

0 — 1.0

I-93 / 99

28 / I-93

O'Brien Hwy.

Paul Revere Park

N. Pt. Park

Martha

Cambridge St.

Beacon St.

Boston Common

Boston

Charles St.

Comm. Ave.

Boylston St.

Land Blvd.

Museum of Science

Longfellow Bridge

First St.

Third St.

Binney

Main St.

Esplanade

Storrow Dr.

Charles River

Mass. Ave.

Hampshire

Windsor

M.I.T.

Harvard Bridge

Prospect St.

Cambridge St.

Broadway

2A

Vassel St.

Memorial Dr.

Brookline Ave.

Emerald Necklace Greenway (Chap. 46)

2A

Cambridge

Harvard Univ.

Mass. Ave.

Western Ave.

River St.

Brookline St.

Storrow Dr.

Boston Univ.

I-90

Park Dr.

Memorial Dr.

Soldiers Field Rd.

N. Harvard St.

Cambridge St.

Western Ave.

exit 18

Comm. Ave.

St. Paul St.

20

Beacon St.

Brighton Ave.

30

Harvard St.

Winchester St.

Brattle St.

Mt. Auburn St.

Soldiers Field Rd.

Greenough

Eliot Bridge

P

Everet St.

Western Ave.

Allston

Warren

2

Coolidge Ave.

Mt. Auburn Cemetery

Grove St.

N. Harvard St.

I-90

N. Beacon St.

Cambridge St.

Market

30

Alewife Area Bike Paths (Chap. 40)

16

Belmont St.

Mt. Auburn St. trail construction

Arlington St.

Arsenal St.

Greenough

20

Arlington

Parsons

Washington St.

16

Watertown Greenway

▼ continued at top of next page ▼

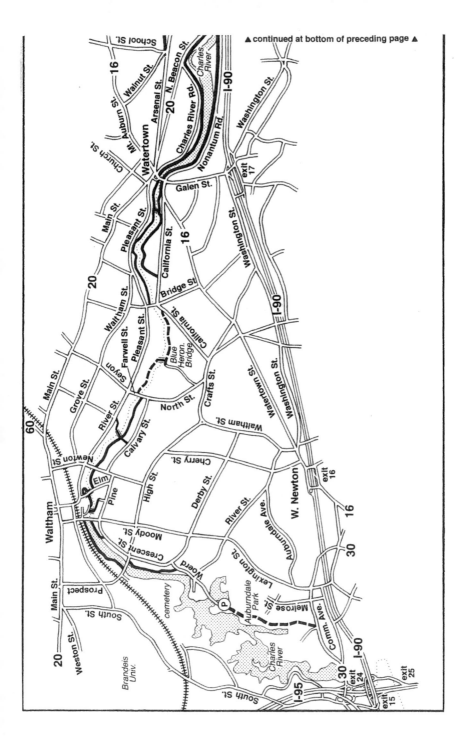

177

and curving over the water as it passes under the **Longfellow Bridge** (4.5 miles). Follow it beside Cambridge Pkwy. to **Land Blvd.** (5.0 miles) then, utilizing sidewalks, turn right at Land and right at **O'Brien Hwy./Rte. 28** to cross the river at the **Museum of Science** (5.2 miles).

Note that another bike path continues east from the O'Brien Hwy. at Museum Way. It begins in **North Point Park**, crosses the spectacular North Bank Bridge over railroad tracks and under the Zakim Bridge/**I-93**, and links **Paul Revere Park** and the Charlestown Bridge/**Rte. 99**.

Returning west on the main loop, turn right on the path beside **Storrow Dr.** along the south side of the river. It passes under the Longfellow Bridge at **Cambridge St.** (5.9 miles) and enters the **Esplanade** where tree-covered paths and arched bridges can be busy with walkers so bicycling is restricted to a designated route. The path continues under the **Harvard Bridge/Mass. Ave.** (7.1 miles), straightens at a corridor of trees, and diverts on a boardwalk under the B.U. Bridge (8.2 miles). It follows Soldiers Field Rd. for the remaining 2.5 miles utilizing crosswalks at **Cambridge St.** (9.1 miles), **Western Ave.** (9.3 miles), and **N. Harvard St.** (9.8 miles) and the Eliot Bridge underpass near the trailhead.

A 7.3-mile loop heads upstream from this parking lot to Watertown Sq. Continuing west beside Soldiers Field Rd., it winds through lawns and wooded areas past the Arsenal St. Bridge (1.2 miles) to **N. Beacon St./Rte. 20** (2.0 miles), then follows the edge of **Nonantum Rd.** to **Galen St./Rte. 16** (3.5 miles). Keeping right, cross the river at Watertown Sq. and return eastward on a stone dust path which connects a paved trail along **Charles River Rd.** Turn right on another path beside **N. Beacon St.** (4.7 miles), left before the river alongside **Greenough Blvd.** (5.1 miles), right at Arsenal St. (5.7 miles), left again on Greenough, then cross the Eliot Bridge to return to the trailhead (7.3 miles).

The Charles River Greenway extends for 5.5 miles (one way) beyond Watertown Sq. including several on-road sections. Beginning across Rte. 16 from Nonantum Rd., it forks right at **California St.** with an unpaved surface, passes a dam and the Thompson Footbridge, and follows a boardwalk through a low area. Emerging at California St. in Newton (1.0 mile), turn right, cross **Bridge St.**, and find the greenway ahead on the right. It descends into woods, crosses more boardwalks and the magnificent **Blue Heron Bridge** (1.6 miles) over the river, then hits **Farwell St.** (1.9 miles) in Waltham. Turn left, cross back over the Charles, and find the next segment on the right. Paved, it intersects a side trail and pedestrian bridge over the river, crosses **Newton St.** (2.7 miles), and then reaches **Elm St.** (2.9 miles). Turn right on Elm, cross the river, then turn right and follow the greenway under the Elm St. bridge and onto a boardwalk above the water. At the end, continue upstream on Landry Way and cross busy **Moody St.** (3.2 miles).

Continuing along the river, turn left on **Prospect St.** (3.8 miles), cross the bridge, then turn right at the Watch Factory Riverwalk and follow its painted blue line between a mill building and the water. Enter woods at the end on an unpaved path to **Woerd Ave.** (4.2 miles), then turn right (south) and follow Woerd, which becomes Forest Grove Rd., uphill to the end (4.7 miles). The last leg is a woodsy trail which descends with a gravelly surface into Newton, flattens with smoother riding near **Auburndale Park**, and ends at **Commonwealth Ave./Rte. 30** (5.5 miles).

BACKGROUND:

The banks of the Charles River became parkland in 1889 and, after the Charles River Dam was built in 1910, were enhanced in 1936. The reservation's original bike path, the state's oldest, was built in 1960 and dedicated to cardiologist and exercise advocate Dr. Paul Dudley White. Additional path construction began in the 1990's to link greenspaces in Boston, Waltham, and Newton.

DRIVING DIRECTIONS:

From I-90 (Mass. Tpke.): Take Exit 18 following signs for Cambridge/Somerville off the ramp. Turn left (west) at the first traffic signal on Soldiers Field Rd. toward Arlington and Newton and continue westbound for 1 mile (keeping left at the fork ahead). Look for trailhead parking lots on the right.

46 Emerald Necklace Greenway

Boston

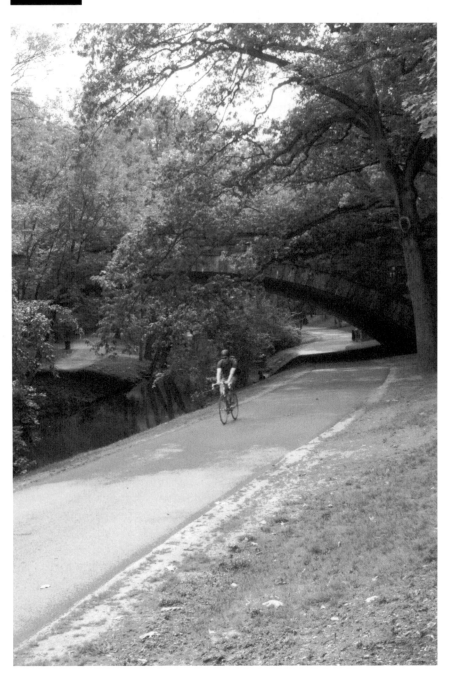

LENGTH: 18 miles
SURFACE: mostly paved
TERRAIN: mostly flat, with hillier terrain at parks

Boston's *Emerald Necklace* of parks and greenways adorns the outskirts of the city with miles of car-free biking, but a few missing links require on-road connections.

RULES & SAFETY:

• Bicycling and in-line skating are not permitted on the trail that circles the western side of Jamaica Pond.

• Note that bicyclists and pedestrians have separate designated trails in some areas.

• Picnicking is not permitted at the Arnold Arboretum.

• Bicyclists should yield to pedestrians.

• Keep to the right, pass on the left, and alert others (*"On your left..."*) when approaching from behind.

• Be especially cautious in the presence of children and pets since their movements can be unpredictable.

• Step off the trail when stopped so others can pass.

• Stop at road intersections and remember that drivers might not be aware of your presence. Car traffic can be busy and fast so make use of crosswalks and signals where they are available.

• Pets must be leashed and their wastes removed.

• The parks are open daily from sunrise to sunset.

• Watch for additional information posted at trailheads.

ORIENTATION:

This collection of parklands provides segments of bike paths which are not contiguous. Biking between the parks requires riding on busy roads and is not recommended.

The easiest, flattest biking lies along the former rail line in Southwest Corridor Park which also has the safest road crossings. Olmsted Park and the Riverway have gentle terrain but also numerous road crossings which are not pedestrian friendly. Both Arnold Arboretum and Franklin Park have hilly terrain and few road intersections.

Olmsted Park and Franklin Park have trailhead

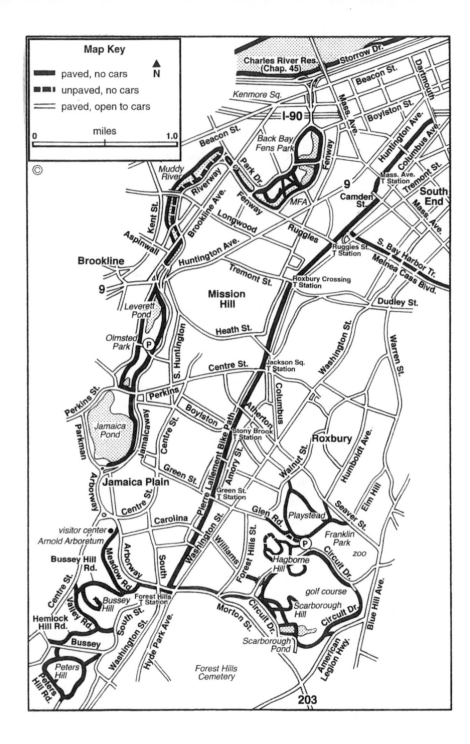

parking lots but Arnold Arboretum and Southwest Corridor Park rely mostly on roadside parking.

TRAIL DESCRIPTION:

Beginning at the Willow Pond Rd. trailhead at **Olmsted Park**, bike paths head north through a slender greenspace for about 2.5 miles. After passing **Leverett Pond** cyclists must carefully cross **Huntington Ave./Rte. 9** (0.6 miles) to reach the Riverway Park, continuing along River Rd. and a paved trail beside **Brookline Ave.** Before crossing a bridge over **Muddy River**, cross the street and veer left on the next section of trail which continues downstream along the tranquil flow as it curves beneath arched bridges and tall shade trees. The trail passes under **Longwood Ave.** near the midpoint and ends at **Park Dr.** (1.7 miles) near the intersection of the **Riverway** and the **Fenway.** Cross Park Dr. at the traffic signal to continue on trails extending for another 0.8 miles through the **Back Bay Fens Park** which follows the river with landscaped areas, playing fields, and community gardens. More paved trails at the **Charles River Reservation** (Chapter 45) await nearby.

Heading south from the Willow Pond Rd. trailhead, a mile of trail parallels the **Jamaica Way** to the southern tip of **Jamaica Pond.** Note that bicyclists and pedestrians have separate trails designated along much of this distance and that the trail circling the pond's western shore is off-limits to biking. This is a popular area for walkers so use caution.

Arnold Arboretum lies three quarters of a mile to the south along the **Arborway** and has about 3.5 miles of gated paved roads exploring a beautiful landscape of diverse trees and shrubs. Begin at its northern entrance near the **visitor center** on **Meadow Rd.** which turns slowly through a flat area for a half-mile, then turn right on **Bussey Hill Rd.** which climbs 200' **Bussey Hill** for a view. Continuing south, return halfway down the slope, turn left at the next two intersections, and follow **Valley Rd.** downward for a third of a mile between two hills. Turn right at the bottom on **Hemlock Hill Rd.** and ride for 0.4 miles through an area of evergreens to the end, then cross **Bussey St.** to reach the mile-long loop of **Peters Hill Rd.** A path inside this loop climbs **Peters Hill** for a view of the city skyline.

    Franklin Park is about a mile to the east and holds over 4 miles of car-free biking. Near the **Circuit Dr.** trailhead, a 0.9-mile loop explores the relatively flat terrain of the **Playstead**, an area of athletic fields beside the **Franklin Park Zoo.** Across Circuit Dr., a 2-mile loop circles a **golf course** in hillier terrain with pretty scenery near **Scarborough Pond** and a strenuous side trip up the half-mile of switchbacks to the top of **Scarborough Hill.** Closer to the trailhead, a cluster of both paved and unpaved trails at **Hagborne Hill** explores a woodsy area of the park known as the Wilderness.

    Southwest Corridor Park and its **Pierre Lallement Bike Path** extend northeastward from the **Forest Hills T Station** to Copley Sq. along a flat, 3.8-mile strip of greenspace with separate surfaces designated for bicyclists and pedestrians along much of the way. T stations, located at roughly half-mile increments, together with road intersections provide useful landmarks. The path parallels the Orange Line, crossing it at large earthen "decks" which are landscaped with plantings. After the **Ruggles St. T Station** (2.7 miles), it intersects the **S. Bay Harbor Tr.** which heads east along **Melnea Cass Blvd.** for 1.3 miles to I-93. Continuing inbound, the Pierre Lallement skirts athletic facilities and emerges on **Camden St.** where cyclists turn left and look for the next section of trail on the right. Just ahead, the crossing of **Mass. Ave.** (3.3 miles) requires caution but links the last half-mile to **Dartmouth St.** which is a peaceful ride past urban gardens in a residential area.

BACKGROUND:

    Boston's so-called *Emerald Necklace* of parks and parkways was conceived in the late 1800's to surround the city with greenspace so that residents could find relief from the stress and confinement of urban living. Frederick Law Olmsted, considered to be the father of landscape architecture, led this effort and designed many of Boston's parks including the Back Bay Fens, the Riverway, the Arnold Arboretum, and Franklin Park. He also designed New York's Central Park and San Fransisco's Golden Gate Park.

A visionary urban planner, Olmsted reshaped these lands to be both naturally beautiful and useful for recreation and transportation. At the Riverway, he directed the Muddy River to be rerouted and its banks to be carefully sculpted to suit the carriage roads running alongside. At Franklin Park, which is named after native Bostonian Benjamin Franklin, Olmsted created the "Playstead" for organized events and a separate "Country Park" for rural scenery.

Southwest Corridor Park originated a hundred years later. When construction of I-95 through Boston was halted in this area by community opposition, efforts turned to securing the route for a new linear park and transit line. Where over 500 homes and businesses had been demolished for the highway, a series of recreation facilities, gardens, and Orange Line T stations were dedicated in 1988. The bike path is named for Pierre Lallement who is credited with bringing the pedal bicycle to America.

DRIVING DIRECTIONS:

- **Riverway from I-95/Rte. 128:** Take Exit 20A for Rte. 9 east. After 7 miles, turn right on Rte. 1 south (the Jamaicaway) and drive for a half-mile, turn right on Willow Pond Rd., and turn immediately right at the parking lot.

- **Arboretum from I-95/Rte. 128:** Take Exit 20A for Rte. 9 east. After 7 miles, turn right on Rte. 1 south (the Jamaicaway) and drive for 1.8 miles to a second traffic circle, then take Rte. 203 east (the Arborway). Park beside the road at the gate one tenth of a mile ahead.

- **Franklin Park from I-93:** Take Exit 15 and follow Columbia Rd. west for 2.2 miles. Cross Blue Hill Ave. and continue on Circuit Dr., then look for the parking lot on the right after a half-mile near the Franklin Park Zoo.

- **Southwest Corridor Park from I-93:** Take Exit 15 and follow Columbia Rd. west for 2.2 miles. Cross Blue Hill Ave. and continue on Circuit Dr. for 1.5 miles to a rotary, then take the first exit following a sign to Forest Hills. Turn left at the next traffic signal on Washington St. and then turn right at the parking lot.

TOILETS:

Arnold Arboretum visitor ctr., Southwest Corridor Park's T stations, Jamaica Pond (seasonal), Franklin Park golf clubhouse (seasonal).

Millenium Park
Boston

LENGTH: 4 miles, plus 1.5 miles of adjoining unpaved trails
SURFACE: paved
TERRAIN: moderate slopes

This cluster of bike paths circles playing fields in a grassy, hilltop setting beside the Charles River.

RULES & SAFETY:
- Bicyclists should yield to pedestrians.
- Keep to the right, pass on the left, and alert others (*"On your left..."*) when approaching from behind.
- Be especially cautious in the presence of children and pets since their movements can be unpredictable.
- Step off the trail when stopped so others can pass.
- Do not ride off the trail surfaces.
- Pets must be leashed and their wastes removed.
- The park is open from dawn to dusk.
- Watch for additional information posted at trailheads.

ORIENTATION:
The trails form concentric loops around a hill and the open surroundings assist visitors in finding their way. The innermost and outermost loops are fairly flat while the connecting trails are sloped. The main parking lot at the top of the hill is the park's focal point.

TRAIL DESCRIPTION:
Skyline Loop is a relatively flat 0.6-mile ride around playing fields at the top of the hill with a picnic area at the western end and distant views in all directions. The 1.4-mile **Millenium Park Tr.** follows the park periphery at the base of the hill with more sheltered conditions and natural scenery along **Sawmill Brook** and the **Charles River**. The mid-level, 1.1-mile **Mezzanine Loop** encounters small slopes as it circles the hill with good views of both the horizon and the natural scenery bordering the park. Numerous connecting

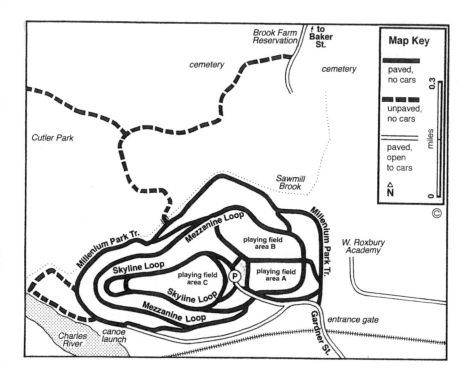

trails hold bigger climbs and descents between these loops.

Heading north, a bridge over **Sawmill Brook** serves unpaved trails extending through woods to **Brook Farm Reservation** off Baker St. and to Wells Ave. Narrower, bumpier conditions make them more challenging to ride.

BACKGROUND:

Millenium Park, completed in 2000, was built upon the former Gardner St. landfill. The park is owned and managed by the city of Boston and its bike paths, playing fields, playground, and canoe launch on the Charles River attract many visitors on sunny weekends.

DRIVING DIRECTIONS:

From I-95/Rte. 128, take Exit 16A and follow Rte. 109 east for 2.5 miles. After crossing the Charles River at the Boston city limits, turn left at a traffic signal on VFW Pkwy., continue for a quarter-mile to another traffic signal, then turn left on Gardner St. Find the park entrance at the end of the road and park at the top of the hill.

TOILETS:

seasonal near the playground at the main parking lot

48 Bay Colony Rail-Trail
Needham

LENGTH: 1.6 miles
SURFACE: stone dust
TERRAIN: flat

This initial segment of the Bay Colony is a worthy first step, a green connection between conservation areas and a peaceful place for biking with young children.

RULES & SAFETY:

- Bicyclists should yield to pedestrians.
- Keep to the right, pass on the left, and alert others (*"On your left..."*) when approaching from behind.
- Dogs must be leashed and their wastes removed.
- Step off the trail when stopped to avoid blocking others.
- Respect nearby residents by keeping noise levels low.
- Visibility at the two road crossings is limited, so remember that drivers might not be aware of your presence.
- The trail is open from dawn until dusk.

ORIENTATION:

Access to the trail is limited to two roads near the western end and, secondarily, to the rougher-surfaced trails of the Needham Town Forest at the eastern end. Both road intersections are well marked by signs and crosswalks.

TRAIL DESCRIPTION:

Beginning at the entrance to the Trustees of Reservation's trailhead on **Fisher St.**, the rail-trail's smooth, stone dust surface extends in two directions. To the west, a 0.3-mile ride reaches a peaceful overlook at the edge of the **Charles River** with southerly views across the broad meadow at **Charles River Peninsula**. To the east, a 1.3-mile segment starts with the crossings of Fisher St. and **Charles River St.**, joins the open corridor of a powerline for a short distance, then bends northeastward through bedrock cuts at the edge of **Needham Town Forest** where hiking and

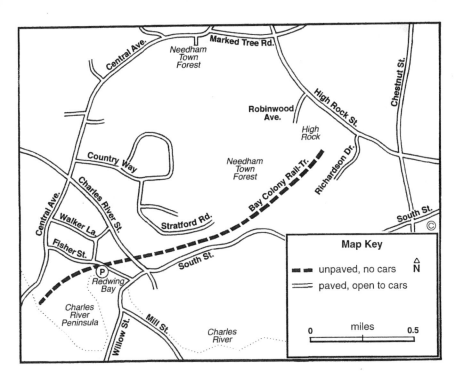

mountain biking paths lead into a wooded terrain of rock outcroppings. The rail-trail dead-ends at a fence before reaching an underpass at **High Rock Rd.**

BACKGROUND:

This rail line was built in the 1850's to haul Needham gravel for filling Boston's Back Bay, was extended to Woonsocket, RI in 1863, and saw its last freight train in 2008. Planning for a rail-trail began a few years later and Needham celebrated the opening of this section in 2016. The trail is envisioned to extend southwest into Dover and Medfield and northeast to the station at Needham Junction.

DRIVING DIRECTIONS:

From I-95, take Exit 17 and follow Rte. 135 west for 0.7 miles to a four-way intersection. Turn left on South St. and continue for 2.5 miles, then turn right on Fisher St. and watch for the entrance to the Charles River Peninsula's trailhead 0.1 miles ahead on the left, just before the rail-trail.

ADDITIONAL INFORMATION:

Bay Colony Rail Trail Association, baycolonyrailtrail.org
Needham Parks & Recreation Dept., (781) 455-7550 x3

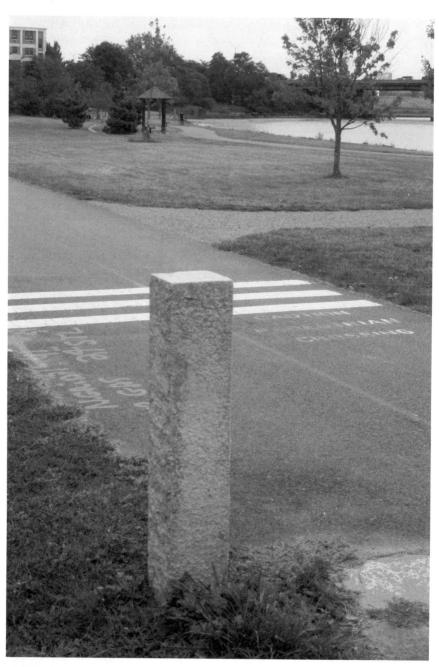

LENGTH: 6 miles including side loops
SURFACE: paved
TERRAIN: flat

Amid busy roads at Boston's southern bounds, this newly expanded rail-trail connects neighborhoods, natural scenery, and local parks along the Neponset River.

RULES & SAFETY:
- Bicyclists should yield to pedestrians.
- Keep to the right, pass on the left, and alert others (*"On your left..."*) when approaching from behind.
- Be especially cautious in the presence of children and pets since their movements can be unpredictable.
- Step off the trail when stopped so others can pass.
- Stop at road intersections and remember that drivers might not be aware of your presence.
- Pets must be leashed and their wastes removed.
- The area is open from dawn until dusk.

ORIENTATION:
The Neponset River Tr. is a rail-trail (and rail-with-trail) for most of its length and joins secondary trails at several parks along the way. Names of intersecting roads, which are few, are posted to assist visitors in determining their location. Pope John Paul II Park is the best point and additional parking is available nearby at the end of Hallet St.

TRAIL DESCRIPTION:
Begin at **Pope John Paul II Park** where 1.3 miles of paved paths loop through landscaped grounds overlooking the **Neponset River**. Downstream to the northeast (turning left when leaving the parking lot), 0.4 miles of trail follow the river under **Rte. 3A** to **Taylor St.** where an additional half-mile paved loop explores **Finnigan Park**. Nearby, **Tenean Beach** on **Conley St.** is reached after 0.3 miles of riding along residential streets and offers a northern view of Boston Harbor and the city skyline.

Heading upstream to the southwest (right when leaving the parking lot) from Pope John Paul II Park, 3.3

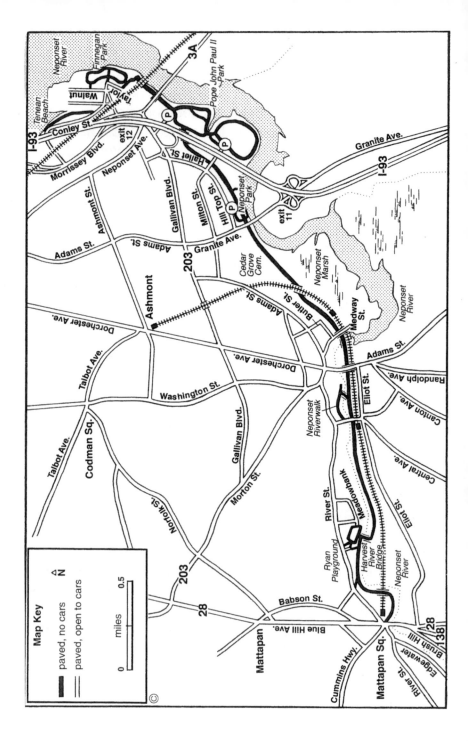

miles of rail-trail start by skirting a playing field, passing under **I-93**, and intersecting **Hallet St.** (0.4 miles). The trail reaches **Neponset Park** (0.6 miles) where drinking water is available and benches enjoy another view of the river, then crosses **Granite St.** (0.7 miles) at a signaled crosswalk.

Here it enters quieter surroundings between Cedar Grove Cemetery and an open vista of **Neponset Marsh**. Continuing under the Ashmont-Mattapan rail line (1.2 miles), the trail parallels the tracks past a station at **Butler St.**, across the river (1.6 miles) and the Milton town line, under **Adams St.** (1.7 miles) near Dorchester's Lower Mills, and along the riverbank to **Central Ave.** (2.0 miles).

The final leg enters woods and eventually turns away from the tracks to cross the Neponset on the magnificent **Harvest River Bridge** (2.7 miles) near an open field at **Ryan Playground**. Continuing upstream in Mattapan, it intersects side trails branching to **River St.**, gradually rises on a high bridge over the rail line (3.0 miles), and circles Mattapan Station before ending at **Blue Hill Ave.** (3.3 miles).

BACKGROUND:

The Neponset River Tr. follows the former Dorchester & Milton Branch Railroad which opened in 1847 and operated until 1959 under the Old Colony Railroad. The state acquired the right of way in 1992 in order to link other properties including the former Hallet St. landfill and the former Neponset Drive-In Theatre which now comprise Pope John Paul II Park. The trail opened between Taylor St. and Central Ave. in 2002 and reached Mattapan Sq. in 2017.

Nepunset, a Native American name, means "Harvest River."

DRIVING DIRECTIONS:

• **Pope John Paul II Park from I-93 northbound:** Take Exit 11, turn right on Granite Ave., and drive for 0.4 miles. Turn right on Hilltop St. and continue for 0.6 miles, turn right on Gallivan Blvd. and continue for 0.1 mile, then turn right at the park entrance (passing under I-93).

• **Pope John Paul II Park from I-93 southbound:** Take Exit 12 and continue for 0.1 mile off the ramp, then turn right at the park entrance (passing under I-93).

TOILETS:

Pope John Paul II Park, Neponset Park

50 Harborwalk Trail
Boston

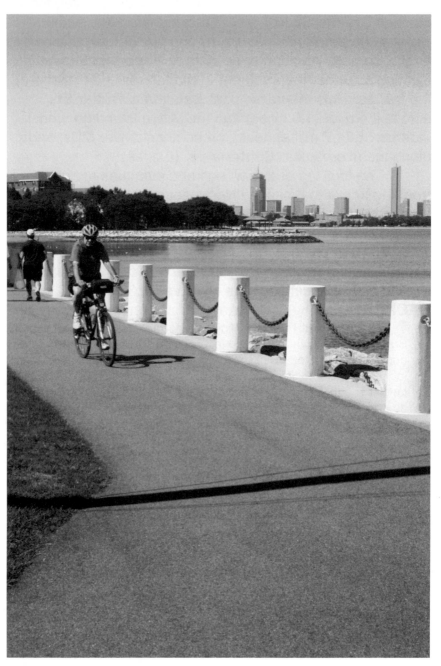

LENGTH: 4.7 miles
SURFACE: paved
TERRAIN: flat
NOTE: busy with pedestrians in warm weather

Sightseers will love this waterfront view of the harbor, airport, and a 5-mile string of beaches, parks, and landmarks.
RULES & SAFETY:
• Bicyclists should yield to pedestrians.

• Bicycling is not permitted at Castle Island and the causeway surrounding Pleasure Bay, which are open only to pedestrians as posted by signs.

• During warm weather when the beaches are crowded, bicyclists should plan on extra slow speeds and expect to share the pathway with large numbers of pedestrians.

• Keep to the right, pass on the left, and alert others (*"On your left..."*) when approaching from behind.

• Use extra caution in the presence of children and pets since their movements can be unpredictable.

• Pets must be leashed and their wastes removed.

• Watch for signs with additional regulations.

• Note that the pathway's exposed location makes it vulnerable to wind and weather.
ORIENTATION:
This route's shoreline location allows easy navigating and intersects no roads, with the exception of Carson Beach's parking lot access points. Parking is provided at points along the way but is not always available during the warm season when crowds of people use the beaches.

Wind can frequently be a factor. Note its direction and remember that starting your ride heading into the wind allows the return trip to be in the easier, downwind direction.
TRAIL DESCRIPTION:
Beginning at the trail's northern end at **Castle Island**, follow the broad, tree-lined pathway beside **Day Blvd.** along the shore of **Pleasure Bay**. (Note that bicycling is not permitted on the paths that surround the fort and on the

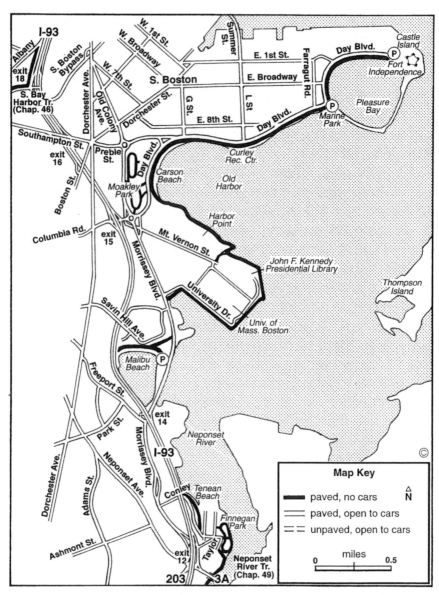

causeway around the bay.) Curving south with the beach, the Harborwalk Tr. reaches a parking lot at **Marine Park** (0.7 miles) and turns west (right) past several yacht clubs, more beach, and the **Curley Recreation Center**. Near the 2-mile-mark it bends back to the south circling **Old Harbor** along crescent-shaped **Carson Beach** with shade trees and benches for those who want to linger. Across the street, a mile of paved trails surround the fields of **Moakley Park**.

Near its midpoint (2.4 miles), the Harborwalk Tr. separates from Day Blvd., leaving the beaches and straightening along the top of a seawall for its remaining distance. Fork left (away from the road) just after the bath house and parking lots at Carson Beach and continue southeastward into quieter surroundings near the **Harbor Point** neighborhood where a mile-long, tree-shaded promenade offers benches and pavilions overlooking the water. Near the end of **Mount Vernon St.**, the trail curves around a small point and cove and then reaches the grounds of the **John F. Kennedy Presidential Library** (3.6 miles) where it turns south. A difference in elevation separates the trail from parallel **University Dr.** and lends a more secluded atmosphere near the **University of Massachusetts Boston**, with side trails rising to connect the campus. After turning northwest, the trail ends at a sidewalk along **Morrissey Blvd.** (4.7 miles).

BACKGROUND:

Castle Island's strategic location on the harbor first established it as a military post in 1634. Fort Independence, built between 1834 and 1851, still stands as a relic at the island's high point and is open for viewing in the summer months. (Hours are posted at the entrance.) The island also served as a prison and a quarantine station. It was joined to the mainland in 1892 as part of a grand design by Frederick Law Olmsted, father of landscape architecture, to surround Boston with parks and greenspace. More recently, efforts to provide better access to the city's shoreline created this section of the Harborwalk, a multi-use trail utilizing DCR's Old Harbor and Dorchester Shores reservations, which is envisioned to extend southward to the Neponset River Tr. (Chapter 49).

DRIVING DIRECTIONS:

From I-93 (Southeast Expressway): Take Exit 15 and turn east on Columbia Rd. At the rotary (Columbus Circle), follow signs for Day Blvd. and continue for 2.5 miles along the shoreline to the end at Castle Island, or watch for other available parking spaces along the way.

TOILETS:

During the warm season: swimming beaches, Castle Island

Bare Cove Park, Great Esker Park
Hingham, Weymouth

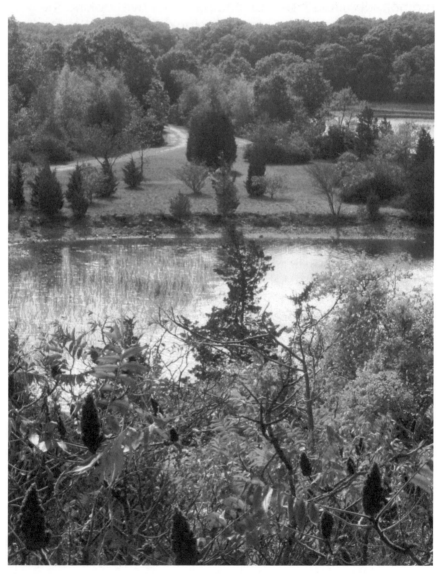

LENGTH: 8.1 miles in two separate areas
SURFACE: mostly paved
TERRAIN: slopes are small at Bare Cove, big at Great Esker

Although they are not connected, these town-owned parklands surround an estuary with acres of greenspace, beautiful water views, and a variety of terrain.

RULES & SAFETY:
- Bicyclists should yield to pedestrians.
- Keep to the right, pass on the left, and alert others (*"On your left..."*) when approaching from behind.
- Be especially cautious in the presence of children and pets since their movements can be unpredictable.
- Swimming is not permitted.
- Pets should be leashed and their wastes removed.
- Watch for additional information posted at trailheads.

ORIENTATION:
Bare Cove Park and Great Esker Park are separate properties on opposite sides of the Back River and are not easily linked by bicycle. Trailhead parking is available on both sides so plan to visit each park separately.

The two parks have noticeably different characters. Bare Cove Park's paved trail network gets greater visitation and has gentle terrain, many views from open areas, and helpful amenities such as intersection signs, maps posted at numerous locations, and mowed grass borders. Great Esker's one road has equally good views with bigger hills and plenty of solitude.

TRAIL DESCRIPTION:
Bare Cove Park in Hingham offers 5.5 miles of paved, car-free biking. Beginning at the **Bare Cove Park Dr.** trailhead, **Bare Cove Path** offers a broad swathe of pavement which is often busy with dog walkers, so pedal cautiously. Heading west, the trail stays straight at the first intersection, reaches its first water view at **Beal Cove** after a quarter-mile, then rolls with gentle slopes along the shoreline to the edge of the **Weymouth Back River** where it turns

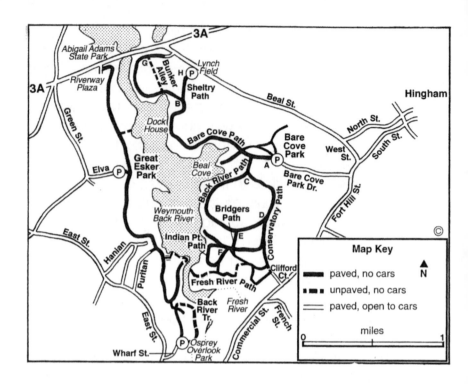

north at the **Dock House** (0.7 miles). After intersecting
Sheltry Path (1.0 mile) which forks right to link another
trailhead at **Lynch Field**, Bare Cove Path continues past
shoreline views for another half-mile before turning inland
beside **Rte. 3A** and ending at **Beal St.** (1.7 miles). Gravel-
surfaced **Bunker Alley** offers a shorter, rougher alternative.

   Back River Path heads south from Bare Cove Path
near the main trailhead. It follows high ground along the
shoreline for about a half-mile with views of the water
through trees, then turns inland to intersect other trails. The
adjoining **Conservatory Path** closely follows the park's
eastern boundary for much of its distance. Watch for the
crumbling pavement of **Fresh River Path** to continue along
the park's southern bounds with rougher surfaces in places
and a narrower width. After descending an unpaved slope, it
passes a few residences and traces the edge of wetlands
along the **Fresh River** before ending after 0.9 miles at the
edge of the Back River. Nearby, the **Indian Point Path**

makes a 0.4-mile loop with more river views.

Great Esker Park in Weymouth lies across the river with a strenuous, 2-mile ride along the crest of a 90'-high esker, the tallest in North America, formed by a subglacial streambed during the Ice Age. From the **Elva Rd.** parking lot, follow the paved trail into woods and up the slope to reach the main trail. Turning to the left (north), it extends for 0.8 miles to **Rte. 3A**, first following the top of the esker and then dropping on a big slope which deserves caution since "speed bumps" placed to divert rainwater can be hazardous for bicyclists. At the bottom, turn right on a short, gravel trail to enjoy a wide view of the river. To the right (south), the road extends for 1.2 miles on a scenic trip to the edge of the Back River, rolling for a half-mile along the top of the ridge, descending steeply with a sharp turn past **Puritan Rd.**, then circling a marsh and ending at a point of land beside the water. After 0.9 miles, watch for the intersecting **Back River Tr.** which makes a 0.6-mile, mostly unpaved loop through adjoining **Osprey Overlook Park**.

BACKGROUND:

Bare Cove Park and Great Esker Park were previously military property and served as an ammunition depot for the assembly, storage, and transfer of mines, torpedos, and other supplies during both world wars and the Korean Conflict. After the facility's usefulness declined, Weymouth acquired the land for Great Esker Park in 1967 and Hingham acquired Bare Cove Park in 1972.

DRIVING DIRECTIONS:

From Rte. 3: Take Exit 16A for Rte. 18 north. Drive for 0.8 miles, turn left (north) on Rte. 53 and continue for 3.3 miles, turn right (south) on Rte. 3A, then as follows:

1. To reach Bare Cove Park in Hingham follow Rte. 3A south for 2.8 miles, bear right on Beal St. and drive for 1.3 miles, continue straight on West St. for 0.2 miles, continue straight on Fort Hill St. and take the next right on Bare Cove Park Dr. Park at the end, a half-mile ahead.

2. To reach Great Esker Park in Weymouth follow Rte. 3A for 2.2 miles, turn right on Green St. and drive for 0.6 miles, then turn left on Elva Rd. and park at the end.

52 World's End Reservation
Hingham

LENGTH: 4.3 miles
SURFACE: crushed stone or mowed grass
TERRAIN: gradual slopes

One of the Boston area's prettiest parklands, this peninsula of tree-lined carriage roads, hillside fields, and harbor views is a visual treat.

RULES & SAFETY:

- Bicyclists should yield to pedestrians.
- Keep to the right, pass on the left, and alert others (*"On your left..."*) when approaching from behind.
- Stay on the trails and do not ride across the fields.
- Pets must be leashed and their wastes removed.
- An admission fee is charged at the entrance.

ORIENTATION:

Trail signs are not present but shoreline confines all sides of the reservation and the open landscape will assist newcomers in finding their way. The carriage roads form loops around a series of small hills with flatter options following the shoreline and hillier ones branching inland. Stop at the ranger station for additional information and maps.

TRAIL DESCRIPTION:

Brewer Rd. begins at the **ranger station** and heads north for three quarters of a mile along the peninsula's western shore with a smooth surface of crushed stone. It rises through a hay field on the slope of **Pine Hill** to a view over **Hingham Harbor**, descends briefly, then begins a second incline at **Planter's Hill** where a grassy side trail loops to the summit for another great view. At the end, turn right on grassy **Weir River Rd.** to return to the trailhead on a mostly flat, 0.7-mile route lined with old shade trees.

Cross **the bar**, a 1700's stone causeway, to link the peninsula's outermost land. The main flow of traffic follows

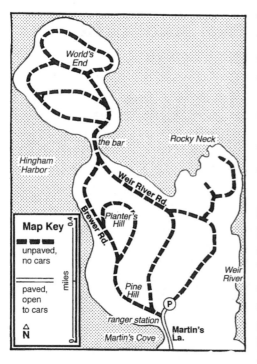

Map Key

- ▬ ▬ ▬ unpaved, no cars
- ═══ paved, open to cars
- △ N
- 0.4 – 0 miles

World's End

the bar

Rocky Neck

Hingham Harbor

Weir River Rd.

Brewer Rd.

Planter's Hill

Pine Hill

Weir River

ranger station

Martin's Cove

Martin's La.

the eastern shore past two trails climbing a hill on the left, then descends to a final intersection at the northernmost loop. Turn hard right to reach **World's End** (1.5 miles from the trailhead).

Rocky Neck, a point of ledge at the park's eastern reach, is about a mile from the trailhead. Follow the trail continuing from the end of the parking lot and ride for a half-mile to an intersection at a row of trees, then turn right and ride for another half-mile over small slopes to the end overlooking the **Weir River**.

BACKGROUND:

After years of agricultural use, this land was destined to become a community of 150 homes in the 1890's when tree-lined carriage roads were established under the direction of renowned landscape architect Frederick Law Olmsted, designer of Boston's Franklin Park and New York's Central Park. The development never materialized and the Trustees of Reservations, the country's oldest private land conservation organization, acquired the property in 1967.

DRIVING DIRECTIONS:

From Rte. 3: Take Exit 14 and follow Rte. 228 north for 5.8 miles. Turn left on Kilby St. and immediately left on Summer St. Drive for a half-mile (crossing Rte. 3A) to a traffic signal at Rockland St., then stay straight on Martin's La. and find the reservation 0.7 miles ahead at the end.

TOILETS:

trailhead parking lot

ADDITIONAL INFORMATION:

The Trustees of Reservations, (978) 921-1944, www.the trustees.org

53 Wompatuck State Park
Hingham, Cohasset, Norwell

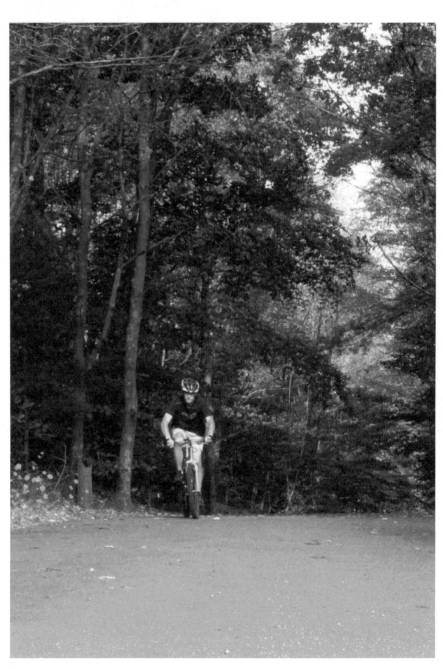

LENGTH: 16 miles
SURFACE: paved
TERRAIN: small hills

Wompatuck's vast, woodsy network of gated roads and rail beds, once part of a World War II-era military depot, are now a popular biking destination. During summer, the 3500-acre park also offers a campground for those who want to spend the night.

RULES & SAFETY:

• Bicyclists should yield to pedestrians.

• Keep to the right, pass on the left, and alert others (*"On your left..."*) when approaching from behind.

• Be especially cautious in the presence of children and pets since their movements can be unpredictable.

• Ride at a safe speed. All routes have two-way traffic and a few have relatively narrow surfaces.

• Do not block trailhead gates when parking since work crews and emergency vehicles always need access.

• Pets should be leashed and their wastes removed.

• Limited hunting is permitted so take appropriate precautions in late fall, the most popular season.

• Watch for additional information posted at trailheads.

ORIENTATION:

This large park's maze of intersections can be confusing so bring a map when exploring for the first time. Maps are also posted on the trails at numerous locations. Unfortunately most of the paved roads and paths remain unnamed but signs at major intersections direct visitors to the park's main trailheads and other destinations. More importantly, numbered markers identify intersections and are displayed on maps to help visitors determine their location. Note that the gated road network includes many dead ends which complicate the task of navigating.

Union St., which is open to cars and offers several options for trailhead parking, forms a 2.5-mile backbone through the center of the park and is accessible only from

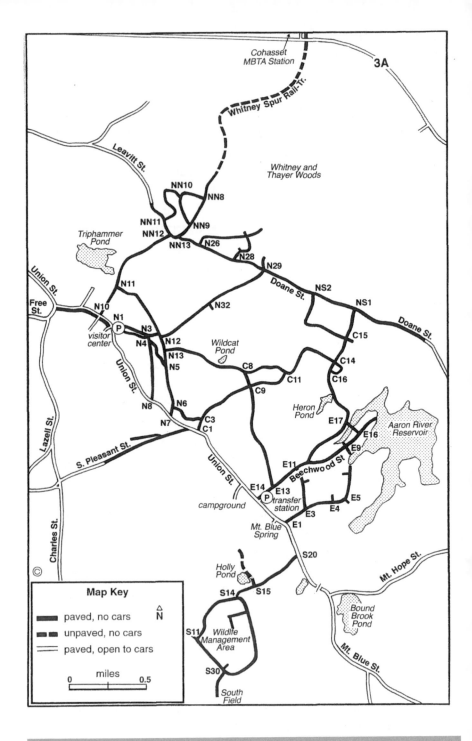

the main entrance. Most of the gated, paved road network lies east of it. Note that Beechwood St. is a gated road that is occasionally used by cars in order to launch non-motorized boats on the Aaron River Reservoir.

The park also has a network of narrower, unpaved trails for mountain biking and hiking which is not displayed on the accompanying map.

TRAIL DESCRIPTION:

Beginning at the main trailhead on **Union St.** in Hingham opposite the state park's **visitor center**, ride past Gate 3 to begin a 5.7-mile narrated loop. Follow the paved road straight past intersection **N3** to intersection **N12** (0.3 miles) and turn left (north) on a section of old rail line. After the paved surface veers off the rail bed and ends at intersection **N11** (0.7 miles), turn right on another road originating from Union St. and continue east past **Triphammer Pond**, which is not visible, to a meadow at intersection **NN12** (1.2 miles) and **Leavitt St.**

Turn right and keep right again at **NN13** to continue southeast on Leavitt St., which becomes **Doane St.** at the Cohasset town line a half-mile ahead. Crumbling in places, this old road has a remote feel as it rolls with small slopes in a woodsy area of rock outcroppings. It passes several side roads including a righthand short-cut at intersection **N29** (1.8 miles) that returns west to the visitor center, 1.1 miles away.

Continuing on the narrated loop, follow Doane St. to intersection **NS1** (2.5 miles) and turn right at a sign for Aaron River Reservoir. Heading south, this road passes a few wetlands, rolls with more hills, and offers a pretty view of **Heron Pond**. Along the way, a sign at intersection **C14** (2.9 miles) marks another righthand short-cut to the visitor center, 1.7 miles away.

The narrated loop turns left at intersection **E17** (3.3 miles) and crosses an arm of **Aaron River Reservoir** to reach **E16** (3.4 miles) at **Beechwood St.**, an access road to the water from Union St. (Note that non-motorized boats are permitted on the reservoir and that vehicles are occasionally permitted to use Beechwood St. in order to launch boats.) Turn right and ride west on Beechwood, crossing back into Hingham and climbing a few bigger slopes before reaching intersection **E13** (4.1 miles) just before the **transfer station** trailhead parking lot on Union St.

A sign at E13 points the way north to the visitor center, 1.7 miles away. Turning right, the narrated loop narrows on another section of former rail bed and enjoys a slight downslope as it passes through a bedrock cut and snakes through an area of ledge and boulders. Spurs to this rail line are evident branching into woods at several points along the way.

Ride straight through intersection **C9** and then keep left at **C8** (4.8 miles) where the paved surface joins a wider road passing grassy **Wildcat Pond**. It curves through a rocky landscape shaded by woods for a half-mile to intersection **N13** (5.3 miles), where a right turn brings riders back to the start of the loop at **N12** (5.4 miles). Turn left and ride 0.3 miles to return to the main trailhead on Union St. (5.7 miles).

Plenty of other trails branch from this loop. The park's most hilly, curvy, and narrow paved bike path lies close to Union St. and links intersections **C9**, **C3**, and **N6**. This 0.7-mile segment has a more challenging character with several steep pitches, a few sharp turns, and a relatively narrow width so ride at a safe speed and remember that the trail has two-way traffic. It passes a grassy picnic area off Union St. near the midpoint.

The **Whitney Spur Rail-Trail** extends northeastward beyond the park's bounds. Once the primary connection between the former military base's network of rail lines and the main line, this 1.8-mile route has recently been developed as a trail from intersection NN13 at the end of Doane St. to the **Cohasset MBTA** station. The trail is paved for the first half-mile to the park boundary, has a smooth, stone dust surface for the 1.2 miles to **Rte. 3A**, then crosses the busy road at a traffic signal and continues with a paved surface for a short distance to the station. Most of the Whitney Spur's rocky, woodland scenery is preserved in the surrounding **Whitney and Thayer Woods**, a property of the Trustees of Reservations.

Alone at the southern end of the park, another few miles of riding reach into neighboring Norwell on a lesser-traveled road circling the park's **Wildlife Management Area**. (Limited hunting is permitted in this area so take appropriate precautions in fall.) It starts near the southern end of Union St. at intersection **S20** with a hill climb above **Holly Pond** then forks after a half-mile at **S14** in a flat, 1.2-mile loop. A few dead end spurs intersect including one at **S30** which branches to the open area of **South Field**.

BACKGROUND:

This property was occupied by the U.S. Navy during World War II and became the country's primary ammunition storage facility on the North Atlantic. Its complex network of roads and rail lines served over 100 underground bunkers which still lurk in the surrounding woods at a few locations.

When the federal government no longer needed the facility, the state of Massachusetts acquired most of the acreage for a park in 1966 and began developing many of the old roads and rail lines into a network of bike paths in 1973. The park takes its name from a Wompanoag chief who, in 1665, deeded land to English settlers for the establishment of Hingham.

The Wompatuck State Park campground is another attraction and is open from mid-April to mid-October. Reservations are recommended.

DRIVING DIRECTIONS:

From Rte. 3: Take Exit 14 and follow signs for Rte. 228 north. After 3.7 miles, turn right on Free St. and drive for 0.8 miles, then turn right on Union St. and continue for a quarter-mile to the parking lot on the left opposite the visitor center. Be careful not to block trailhead gates.

TOILETS:

visitor center

ADDITIONAL INFORMATION:

Wompatuck State Park, Hingham, (781) 749-7160
Friends of Wompatuck, www.friendsofwompatuck.org
campground reservations: www.reserveamerica.com

54 Pond Meadow Park

Braintree, Weymouth

LENGTH: 2.1 miles
SURFACE: paved
TERRAIN: small hills

This rolling, turning trail circles a pond with no road intersections, making it a popular choice for biking with kids.
RULES & SAFETY:
- This is a one-way (clockwise) loop. A painted dividing line keeps bicyclists to the *left* side and walkers to the right.
- Ride at a safe speed since the trail has slopes, curves, and 8'-width.
- Bicycling is allowed only on the paved trail.
- Pets must be leashed and their wastes removed.
- Wading and swimming in the pond are prohibited.
- The park is open from sunrise to sunset. Note the posted time that the parking lot gates are locked each night.
ORIENTATION:
The trail forms a 1.7-mile loop around the pond with side trails connecting two trailheads, one in Braintree and one in Weymouth. Each side trail is marked by signs.
TRAIL DESCRIPTION:
Beginning at the **Braintree trailhead** and **park office** on **Liberty St.**, follow the trail downhill beside the paved access road to the start of the 1.7-mile loop. Heading left (north), it begins with an abrupt uphill and then descends for 0.3 miles to **Twenty-Acre Pond** where picnic tables overlook the water. The trail returns to woods, climbs a slope, and turns south past **Big Meadow** near the 1-mile mark. Curving through woods, it continues to a T-intersection (1.4 miles) where a side trail leads left (east) to the **Weymouth trailhead** on **Summer St.** Turning right (west), the last leg crosses two bridges over inlet streams before returning to the start of the loop but suffers from the traffic noise of parallel **Rte. 3**.

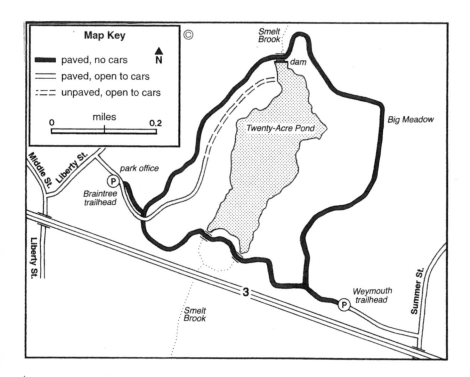

BACKGROUND:

Established in 1976, Pond Meadow Park is a former flood control project now managed by the Weymouth-Braintree Regional Recreation-Conservation District. The paved trail was built in 1984.

DRIVING DIRECTIONS:

Braintree trailhead from Rte. 3: Take Exit 17 and follow signs for Union St. eastbound toward E. Braintree. After 1.2 miles, turn right on Liberty St. and drive 1.1 miles to the park entrance on the left.

Weymouth trailhead from Rte. 3: Follow the directions above but continue on Liberty St. to the end, turn left on Grove St. and drive for 0.5 miles, turn left on West St. and drive for 0.3 miles, turn left on Summer St. and drive for 0.8 miles, then turn left at the park entrance.

TOILETS:

Park Office at the Braintree trailhead

ADDITIONAL INFORMATION:

Pond Meadow Park, (781) 843-7663

55 Hanover Branch Rail-Trail
Rockland-Abington

LENGTH: 2.7 miles
SURFACE: paved
TERRAIN: slight slopes

Spanning the town, Rockland's tree-shaded pathway provides a linear recreation park between the center and outlying natural areas.

RULES & SAFETY:
- Bicyclists should yield to pedestrians
- Keep to the right, pass on the left, and alert others (*"On your left..."*) when approaching from behind.
- Trail users are asked to obey all traffic rules. Stop at road intersections and assume that drivers do not see you.
- Dogs must be leashed and their wastes removed.
- Respect the private property along the trail.
- Note that trailhead parking is currently not provided, and that a 2-hour limit applies to most on-street parking.
- Watch for additional information posted at trailheads.

ORIENTATION:
No official trailhead parking exists so visitors use on-street parking and access the trail from intersecting streets. The trail is identifiable by signs which also function as vehicle barricades. The trail's midpoint near Union St. has the highest elevation and the endpoints have lower elevations.

TRAIL DESCRIPTION:
Heading east from **Union St.** in downtown Rockland, the trail extends for 1.4 miles. It quickly departs the commercial area and passes a residential neighborhood at **Howard St.** and **Vernon St.** (0.3 miles), then descends to **Liberty St./Rte. 123** (0.6 miles) and continues across a parking lot and access road to the **police dept.**

Returning to woods, the remaining 0.8 miles of trail

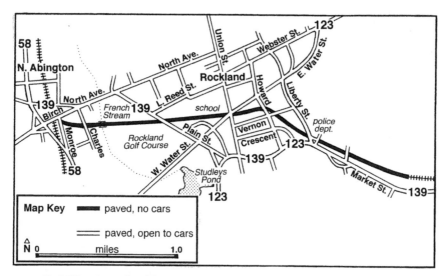

parallel **Market St./Rte. 139** in flat terrain and natural scenery before dead-ending at the Hanover town line (1.4 miles) where railroad tracks remain.

Heading west from Union St., 1.3 miles of trail begin with a downslope past schools and athletic fields, cross **Plain St./Rte. 139** (0.5 miles), and continue past the **Rockland Golf Course** to a bridge over **French Stream** (1.0 mile). The trail enters Abington for its last third of a mile, crossing **Charles St.** and ending at **Monroe St.** (1.3 miles).

BACKGROUND:

This railroad was built in 1868 as the Hanover Branch of the Old Colony Line and operated until 1938. A volunteer effort to transform it to a recreational trail began in 1999 and the rail-trail opened in 2012. In constructing the trail, the town utilized the Iron Horse Preservation Society which salvaged the rails, disposed of the ties, and applied a stone aggregate surface material. Subsequent improvements include an extension to North Abington and asphalt surfacing. A future extension eastward into Hanover is expected.

DRIVING DIRECTIONS;

From Rte. 3 take Exit 13 and follow Rte. 53 north for a half-mile. Turn left (west) on Rte. 123 and drive for 3 miles to a traffic signal (where Rte. 123 turns left on E. Water St.), then continue straight on Webster St. for another 1.7 miles to the end. Turn left on Union St. and look for on-street parking near the rail-trail, which crosses 0.3 miles ahead.

LENGTH: 3.5 miles of bike lane on parkway
SURFACE: paved
TERRAIN: one hill, otherwise gentle

An oasis of nature, this property holds an attractive bike/pedestrian lane on a one-way, lightly traveled parkway circling several large ponds.

RULES & SAFETY:

- Bicyclists should yield to pedestrians.
- Alert others (*"On your left..."*) when passing from behind.
- Be especially cautious in crowded areas and where children or pets are present.
- The loop is one-way in the counter-clockwise direction. The marked bike/pedestrian lane is on the left side of the parkway (inside lane) and the motor vehicle lane is on the right (outside lane). Be alert for occasional passing cars.
- Swimming is prohibited.
- Park only in designated areas.
- The park is open during daylight hours. Note the closing time posted at the entrance gate.

ORIENTATION:

D. W. Field Park's long, thin shape extends from Brockton north into Avon. Oak St. and South St. divide the property into three sections and parking areas, identified by a letter posted on a sign (shown on the map), are helpful points of reference. Parking lot E near Oak St. is the most popular starting point. The parkway encounters one significant hill at the southern end of the loop, otherwise the terrain is gentle.

TRAIL DESCRIPTION:

The 3.5-mile bike/pedestrian lane begins near parking lot **E** which is located off **Oak St.** near **Upper Porter Pond**. Forking right on **East Parkway**, the ride starts with a steep

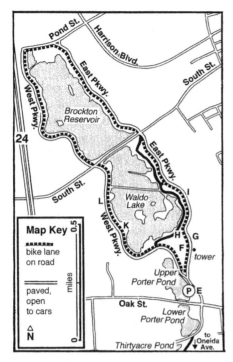

Map Key

bike lane
on road

paved,
open
to cars

△ N

uphill to Brockton's highest point where a 65-foot stone **observation tower** stands above the road. It then descends past a view of **Waldo Lake** and follows its wooded shore north into Avon, crosses **South St.** (0.8 miles), and continues along **Brockton Reservoir** with gentle hills and curves for another 0.6 miles to **Pond St.** (1.4 miles).

Turning left, the loop reverses direction on **West Parkway** with highway noise from **Rte. 24** evident at the start but an otherwise peaceful ride along the reservoir's shoreline. After crossing South St. (2.3 miles), it takes a mile-long, serpentine course along Waldo Lake's western shore before returning to the parking lot E trailhead.

Across Oak St., an aging 0.5-mile paved path extends south from **Lower Porter Pond** with bumpy conditions to connect **Oneida Ave.**

BACKGROUND:

D. W. Field Park is an 800-acre preserve named for a Brockton resident who was prominent in the city's shoe industry during the late 1800's. Known for both his frugality in business and his generosity to the public, Field provided most of the funds to establish the park in the early 1900's and supervised the construction of its parkways, creation of the ponds, and landscaping of the grounds.

DRIVING DIRECTIONS:

From Rte. 24: Take Exit 18B and follow Rte. 27 north for 0.5 miles. Turn right at a traffic signal on Oak St. Ext. and continue for 1.3 miles to the park's main entrance (just after the road passes between two ponds). Note the park's closing time which is posted at the gate.

WWII Veterans Memorial Trail
Mansfield

LENGTH: 1.5 miles
SURFACE: paved
TERRAIN: flat

A safe haven for cyclists of all ages, this short stretch of car-free pavement is the straightest rail-trail in the state.
RULES & SAFETY:
 • Bicyclists should yield to pedestrians.
 • Keep to the right, pass on the left, and alert others (*"On your left..."*) when approaching from behind.
 • Be especially cautious in the presence of children and pets since their movements can be unpredictable.
 • Pets must be leashed and their wastes removed.
ORIENTATION:
The trail's short, straight-line course runs between the Fruit St. trailhead near the Norton town line and downtown Mansfield. Road intersections are limited and are made safe with signs and crosswalks. The trail extends into downtown Mansfield with a marked bike lane through parking lots.
TRAIL DESCRIPTION:
Beginning at the southern endpoint at **Fruit St.**, the trail's straight line extends northwest toward downtown Mansfield. The first mile follows an open corridor in woodsy surroundings interspersed with homes, then the trail comes alongside **Branch St.** for a short distance near the midpoint and crosses **Lincoln Rd.** before returning to woods. Houses appear more frequently on the approach to downtown but trees screen both sides of the trail.
The **World War II Veterans Memorial** stands prominently beside the trail at **East St.** (1.5 miles) along with a plaque describing the railroad's history. A marked bike route follows the original rail line across more streets and several parking lots off **Main St.**

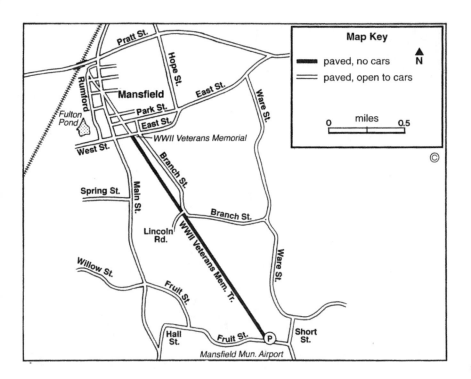

BACKGROUND:

The WWII Veterans Memorial Tr. originated in 1836 as the Old Colony Railroad, a branch line of the Boston & Providence which also runs through Mansfield. Known as one of the straightest rail lines in the state, the Old Colony is remembered for carrying thousands of military personnel during World War II from training at Camp Myles Standish in Taunton to Boston for travel to all parts of the world.

The railroad operated until 1965, lay dormant for decades, and was transformed to a recreational trail in 2004. It is dedicated to the men and women who embarked to the war effort along the route.

DRIVING DIRECTIONS:

From I-95/Rte. 128: Take Exit 7 and follow Rte. 140 south for 1.6 miles. Take the School St. exit toward Mansfield center, then take the first right on Spring St. and continue for a half-mile to the end. Turn right on S. Main St. and continue for another half-mile, then turn left on Fruit St. and look for the trailhead parking lot 1 mile ahead on the left.

57 Myles Standish State Forest
Plymouth-Carver

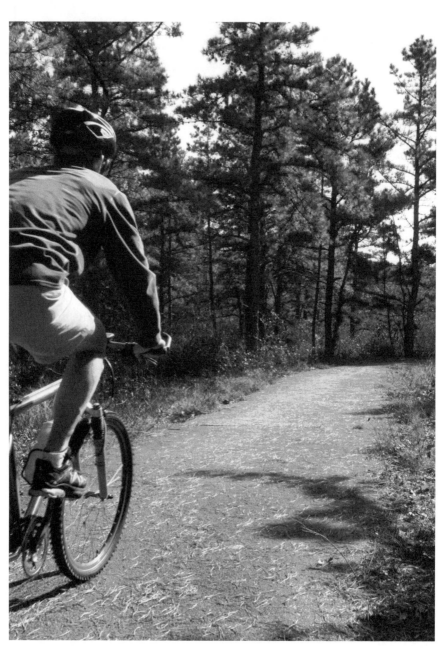

LENGTH: 15.1 miles
SURFACE: paved
TERRAIN: hilly

An expansive paved trail network winds through the distinctive landscape of this 15,000-acre preserve allowing car-free passage between popular campgrounds and freshwater beaches.

RULES & SAFETY:
   • Bicyclists should yield to pedestrians.
   • The two-way trails are curvy, sloped, and relatively narrow so ride at a safe speed and stay alert.
   • Keep to the right, pass on the left, and alert others (*"On your left..."*) when approaching from behind.
   • Use extra caution when children or pets are present.
   • Watch for cracks and bumps in the paved surface and areas of accummulated sand, leaves, and pine needles which can be slippery, especially when wet.
   • Do not block gates when parking since work crews and emergency vehicles always need access.
   • Swimming is permitted only at designated areas which are staffed during the summer season.
   • Hunting is a popular activity and visitors are advised to wear blaze orange clothing in late fall. For safety, all trails are closed on Saturdays and holidays from mid-October until early January and all of deer week of the shotgun season each year. Note that hunting is prohibited by state law on Sundays. Hunting seasons and regulations are posted at many trailheads.
   * Watch for additional rules posted at trailheads.

ORIENTATION:
When planning a biking excursion at Myles Standish realize that the property is vast and that some of the trails are long and hilly. Numbered gates at road crossings (displayed on the map) provide an important means of determining location, and wooden signs display popular destinations at many trail intersections.

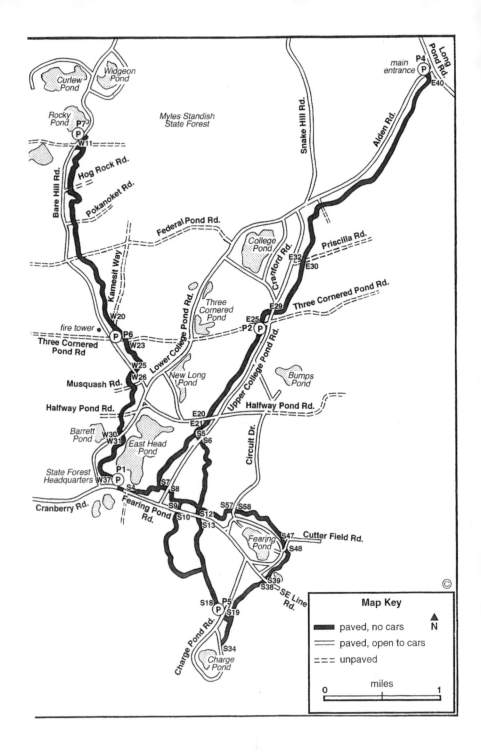

Myles Standish State Forest

Curlew Pond

Widgeon Pond

Rocky Pond
P7
W11

Bare Hill Rd.

Hog Rock Rd.

Pokanoket Rd.

Kamesit Way

Federal Pond Rd.

College Pond

Cranford Rd.

Snake Hill Rd.

main entrance
P4
Long Pond Rd.
E40

Alden Rd.

Priscilla Rd.

E32
E30

Three Cornered Pond Rd.

Three Cornered Pond

E29

E25
P2

fire tower
P6
W20
P
W23
W25
W26

Three Cornered Pond Rd

Lower College Pond Rd.

Musquash Rd.

New Long Pond

Upper College Pond Rd.

Bumps Pond

Halfway Pond Rd.

Halfway Pond Rd.

Barrett Pond
W30
W31

East Head Pond

E20
E21
S5
S6

Circuit Dr.

State Forest Headquarters
P1
W37
S4
S7
S8

Cranberry Rd.

Fearing Pond Rd.

S9
S10
S12
S13

S57
S58

Fearing Pond

S47
S48

Cutter Field Rd.

S39
S38
SE Line Rd.

S18
P5
S19

Charge Pond Rd.

S34

Charge Pond

©

Map Key

▲ N

━━━ paved, no cars

──── paved, open to cars

=== unpaved

0   miles   1

Several parking lots serve the bike paths. Parking Lot #1 (P1) near Forest Headquarters offers toilets and information while most outlying lots have no facilities. Note that trail signs identify trailheads with abbreviations such as *"P2"* for Parking Lot #2. The bridge on Fearing Pond Rd. near Parking Lot #1 and Forest Headquarters is closed to vehicles but open to bicyclists and pedestrians.

TRAIL DESCRIPTIONS:

Beginning at Parking Lot #1 (**P1**) and the Interpretive Center at **Forest Headquarters** on **Fearing Pond Rd.**, the longest paved bike path extends northeastward for 5.7 miles to the state forest's **main entrance**. From the parking lot, turn left on Fearing Pond Rd., cross the bridge, and find the trail on the left at gate **S4** after 0.2 miles. It rises on a slope, levels on a winding course through a pine forest, and then drops on a hill with a sharp, left-hand turn at the bottom.

Here at the 0.6-mile mark it intersects another bike path on the right near gate S7 leading east to Fearing and Charge ponds. Continuing north (straight) at this junction, the trail rolls with ups and downs for 0.8 miles to **Halfway Pond Rd.** (1.4 miles) at gate **E21**, intersecting a second bike path leading to Fearing and Charge ponds along the way near gate **S5**. The paved surface is interrupted for 20 feet as the trail crosses a gas pipeline along this distance.

North of Halfway Pond Rd., the trail flattens for over a mile alongside **Upper College Pond Rd.** with bushes and foliage obscurring the sight of the nearby roadway. It passes Parking Lot #2 (**P2**) at gate **E25** and **Three Cornered Pond Rd.** (2.6 miles), then crosses to the east side of Upper College Pond Rd. and meanders for a half-mile through a more open environment of pitch pines and scrub oaks. Crossing the gravel surface of **Priscilla Rd.** (gates **E30/E32**), the path's final 2.5 miles roll with small hills and weave through woods. It turns eastward beside **Alden Rd.**, crosses a powerline (3.9 miles), and ends at the main entrance on **Long Pond Rd.** (5.7 miles) at gate **E40**.

The two paved trails heading east from this route link

popular picnicking, swimming, and camping locations at the south end of the state forest. From gates **S7/S8**, it is a hilly, 2.8-mile ride around the eastern side of **Fearing Pond** to **Charge Pond**. After crossing **Circuit Dr.** (0.6 miles) at gates **S57/S58**, the trail ascends a few slopes and enjoys a series of descents to **Cutter Field Rd.** (1.4 miles) at gates **S47/S48** near the swimming beach at Fearing Pond. The trail rolls with small hills to **Southeast Line Rd.** (1.8 miles) at gates **S38/S39** then stays flat for the last leg to **Charge Pond Rd.** (2.7 miles) at gate **S34** near Charge Pond.

Just before this endpoint turn right on a trail which drops to gate **S19** and crosses Charge Pond Rd. at Parking Lot #5 (**P5**). (Use caution at this road crossing since the trail descends steeply.) Returning to the northwest, this trail splits after a half-mile and both options intersect **Fearing Pond Rd.**, with the right-hand option being the flattest route. Keeping left at this fork, continue for another mile and cross Fearing Pond Rd. at gates **S9/S10**, then turn left to return to Forest Headquarters 0.9 miles away.

The state forest's hilliest, curviest paved bike path is 4-mile option (one way) heading north from Parking Lot #1. Climbing from gate **W37** above the headquarters building, it weaves through trees and rolls through undulating terrain above **East Head Reservoir**, crosses **Lower College Pond Rd.** (0.8 miles) at gates **W30/31** and tackles more slopes on the way to **Bare Hill Rd.** (1.4 miles) at gates **W25/26**. The trail parallels Bare Hill Rd. for the remaining distance, meeting longer and steeper slopes as it climbs to the forest's highest elevation at the **fire tower** and Parking Lot #6 (**P6**) (1.7 miles). Here it crosses **Three Cornered Pond Rd.** (gate **W23**) and **Kamesit Way** (gate **W20**), levels for a short distance, and makes a half-mile descent to **Federal Pond Rd.** It continues with more ups, downs, and frequent turns including a downhill hair-pin which deserves caution. The trail's last half-mile holds a series of mostly uphill pitches before it emerges at a powerline and drops to Bare Hill Rd. (4.0 miles) at gate **W11** near Parking Lot #7 (**P7**).

BACKGROUND:

Myles Standish State Forest is New England's largest *pine barren* ecosystem, a sandy environment where only low-growing pitch pines, scrub oaks, and other hardy plants can survive. Named for the military leader of Plymouth Colony, it was established in 1916 in one of the first acts of a newly created State Forest Commission. At the time, the land was considered of little value but its ponds and woodlands gradually became a recreation resource and in the 1930's the Civilian Conservation Corps built bath houses, beaches, picnic areas, campgrounds, and roads to suit growing numbers of visitors.

The 15 miles of paved bike paths were built in the 1970's to complement the forest's other summer attractions of campgrounds (reservations recommended) and two day-use swimming beaches. In addition, many more miles of unpaved trails and roads venture into remote areas for mountain biking, horseback riding, and hiking.

The state forest's numerous ponds are *kettle holes* formed at the end of the last ice age when huge blocks of ice broke from a glacier and began to melt, creating depressions which filled with water.

DRIVING DIRECTIONS:

• **From I-495:** Take Exit 2 and follow Rte. 58 north for 2.4 miles. Where Rte. 58 turns sharply left, continue straight on Tremont St. (following a sign to Plymouth) and drive for another 0.8 miles. Turn right on Cranberry Rd., continue for 2.7 miles to a left-hand curve at forest headquarters, and turn right at the Interpretive Center (Parking Lot #1).

• **From Rte. 3 southbound:** Take Exit 5 and follow Long Pond Rd. for 3.6 miles, then turn right at the state forest's main entrance on Alden Rd. and drive for 1.8 miles. Either keep left on Upper College Pond Rd. for 1.1 miles to Parking Lot #2 (on the right), or fork left on Lower College Pond Rd. and look for Parking Lot #1 after 3.6 miles on the left at Forest Headquarters and a sharp, right turn.

• **From Rte. 3 northbound:** Take Exit 3. Turn left on Clark Rd. and drive for 0.4 miles, turn right on Long Pond Rd. and continue for 2 miles, turn left at the main entrance, and follow the above directions.

TOILETS:

Forest Headquarters, and seasonally at other locations.

ADDITIONAL INFORMATION:

Myles Standish State Forest, (508) 866-2526,
www.mass.gov/eea/agencies/dcr/massparks

59 Quequechan River Rail-Tr.
Fall River

LENGTH: 2.6 miles
SURFACE: paved
TERRAIN: flat

This riverbank and lakeshore trail brings welcome recreation and greenspace to the heart of the city, although highway noise is never far away.

RULES & SAFETY:
- Bicyclists should yield to pedestrians.
- Keep to the right, pass on the left, and alert others (*"On your left..."*) when approaching from behind.
- Be especially cautious in the presence of children and pets since their movements can be unpredictable.
- The trail is open from 6:00AM-9:00PM.
- The trail encounters only two road intersections but both deserve extra caution since traffic levels are high. Remember that drivers might not be aware of your presence.
- Pets must be leashed and their wastes removed.

ORIENTATION:
The main trail is 2 miles long with two branches near the western end. Granite posts display destinations at these intersections and maps are located at several points.

TRAIL DESCRIPTION:
Beginning at the entrance to **Britland Park**, the paved path soon reaches a T-intersection. To the left, a quarter-mile of trail extends eastward along playing fields and the **Quequechan River**. To the right, 2 miles of trail begin with a bridge over a channel and then follow a former railroad bed between the river and **I-195**. Ahead on the right, a side trail utilizes a highway underpass to reach **Rodman St.**

Continuing straight, the main trail extends southeastward over more bridges, intersects **Quequechan St.** (0.7 miles from Britland Park), and slips under both I-195

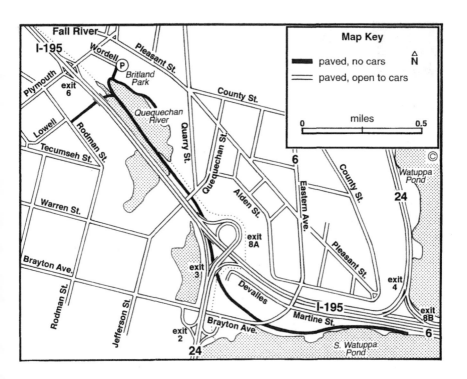

and **Rte. 24** before intersecting 4-lane **Brayton Ave.** (1.3 miles). The last leg follows the shore of **S. Watuppa Pond** with quieter surroundings and a broad view, passing office buildings and businesses along the way before dead-ending near the edge of **Martine St./Rte. 6** (2.0 miles) and I-195.

BACKGROUND:

Fall River takes its name from the Quequechan River, named by the Wompanoag natives for its *"falling water"* which flowed over 8 waterfalls between S. Watuppa Pond and the nearby Taunton River. The Quequechan was dammed in the 1800's to generate power for a thriving textile industry prompting the construction of the Fall River Railroad in 1875. Construction of I-195 in 1965 altered the river's course and initiated years of neglect but creation of the first leg of the rail-trail in 2014 has renewed appreciation for the waterway.

DRIVING DIRECTIONS:

From I-195 take Exit 7, follow Rte. 81 (Plymouth Ave.) north, take the first right on Wordell St., and park at the end.

ADDITIONAL INFORMATION:

City of Fall River, Community Maintenance: (508) 324-2584

225

Saulnier Memorial Bike Trail

New Bedford

LENGTH: 6.8 miles
SURFACE: paved
TERRAIN: flat

These waterfront promenades pass popular beaches and a historic fort at the head of the harbor.

RULES & SAFETY:

• Bicyclists should yield to pedestrians. Watch for separate, designated lanes for bicyclists and pedestrians.

• Keep to the right, pass on the left, and alert others (*"On your left..."*) when approaching from behind.

• The trail can be busy on fairweather days especially near the beaches, so use extra caution.

• The area is exposed to wind and adverse weather.

• Dogs must be leashed and their wastes removed.

• Note that the gate at Ft. Tabor Park is locked at dusk.

ORIENTATION:

Paved trails extend in three directions from Fort Taber Park trailhead: south around the fort, north along the western shore of the peninsula, and north along the eastern shore of the peninsula. Road intersections are scarce but some sections of trail follow roadsides closely.

TRAIL DESCRIPTION:

Begin at **Fort Taber Park** where a cluster of paths explores the landscaped grounds of Fort Rodman with excellent views of Buzzards Bay. Following the perimeter route through this area makes a three-quarter-mile loop along the water and can be extended westward through a natural area bordering a wastewater treatment facility.

A path beside **W. Rodney French Blvd.** continues for over a mile with views across **Clark's Cove**. It narrows between the road and a seawall at **West Beach** and ends beyond **Woodlawn St.** at a hurricane wall. Ahead on the

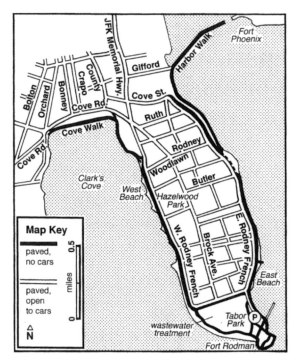

left, 0.9-mile **CoveWalk** extends along the top of this huge stone structure with more water views.

The peninsula's eastern shore offers a similar ride beside **E. Rodney French Blvd.** where a path squeezes past **East Beach**, passes a few fishing piers, and joins a seawall. It's interrupted for a quarter-mile before reaching **Butler St.** and another hurricane barrier, then resumes for a half-mile. Watch on the right for the 1.2-mile **HarborWalk** which climbs to the top of the hurricane barrier and extends into New Bedford Harbor with a great view over the water.

BACKGROUND:

Since the early 1800's, this peninsula has been home to military posts including Fort Taber, built in the late 1850's, and Fort Rodman, built in the 1940's. The area has also provided park space during peacetime since the late 1800's and has been owned by the city of New Bedford since 1992. The bike path is named for Rep. Joseph D. Saulnier, a former city counselor. HarborWalk, opened in 2015, and CoveWalk, opened in 2017, both follow hurricane barrier walls constructed in the 1960's to protect the city from severe storms.

DRIVING DIRECTIONS:

From I-195 take Exit 15 and follow Rte. 18 south for 2.8 miles to a traffic signal at Cove St. (where Rte. 18 ends). Continue straight on W. Rodney French Blvd. and drive for 2 miles, then look for the Fort Taber Park entrance on the right.

TOILETS:

Fort Taber Park, West Beach (seasonal)

61 Phoenix Rail-Trail Mattapoisett Rail-Trail
Fairhaven-Mattapoisett

LENGTH: 4.4 miles, plus 0.9-mile side trail
SURFACE: paved
TERRAIN: slight slopes

Named for nearby Fort Phoenix, this pathway stretches eastward from New Bedford Harbor past saltmarshes, farm fields, and quiet woods along the South Coast.

RULES & SAFETY:
- Bicyclists should yield to pedestrians.
- Keep to the right, pass on the left, and alert others (*"On your left..."*) when approaching from behind.
- Pets must be under control and pet wastes removed.

ORIENTATION:
The trail currently extends from downtown Fairhaven eastward into Mattapoisett with natural surroundings dominating the eastern half. A side trail intersects near the midpoint and curves through woods to a view of Little Bay.

TRAIL DESCRIPTION:
Starting at **Main St.**, the Phoenix Rail-Trail parallels **South St.** and intersects a cluster of residential streets in the first third of a mile. The trail gets greener on the way to **Egypt La.** (0.6 miles), follows conservation land near a flood control wall, then joins the edge of **Drown Blvd.** (1.0 mile) past a shopping center to **Sconticut Neck Rd.** (1.2 miles).

The trail meets the end of **Arsene St.** (1.5 miles) at a **DPW** facility and trailhead parking lot where the 0.9-mile **Little Bay Extension** heads south between huge wind turbines. This side trail curves through woods to **Orchard St.** and offers a worthwhile view of **Little Bay** near the end.

Continuing east, the rail-trail crosses a causeway over the **Nasketucket River** with a view of its marsh and Little Bay. It then rises on a mild slope to a residential area at

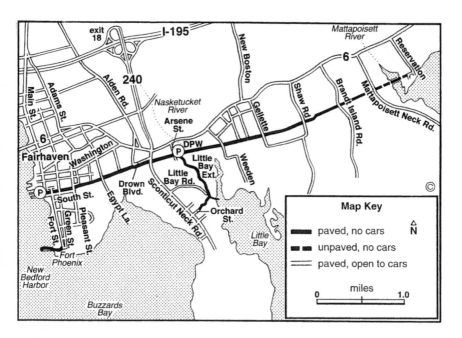

Weeden Rd. (2.1 miles), borders farmland at **Gellette Rd.** (2.6 miles), and hits **Shaw Rd.** (3.1 miles) near the Mattapoisett line. Here the **Mattapoisett Rail-Tr.** continues to **Brandt Island Rd.** (3.5 miles) and **Mattapoisett Neck Rd.** (4.0 miles), then narrows with an unpaved surface over the **Mattapoisett River** to **Reservation Rd.** (4.4 miles).

BACKGROUND:

This route originated in 1854 as the Fairhaven Branch Railroad which operated between New Bedford Harbor and the Cape Cod Branch Railroad in Wareham. After the trains stopped running, Fairhaven acquired its 3.2-mile portion of the line in 1954 and completed trail construction in 1999. Mattapoisett extended the trail in 2009 and is expected to build eastward to Depot St. The trail is envisioned to reach Wareham as part of the South Coast Bikeway.

DRIVING DIRECTIONS:

From I-195, take Exit 18 and follow Rte. 240 south for 1 mile. Turn right on Rte. 6 east and drive for 1.5 miles, then turn left on Main St. before the bridge. Continue south for 0.6 miles to a parking lot on the right just before the intersection of South St., across from the rail-trail.

ADDITIONAL INFORMATION:

South Coast Bikeway: southcoastbikeway.com

62 Cape Cod Canal Bicycle Tr.
Bourne-Sandwich

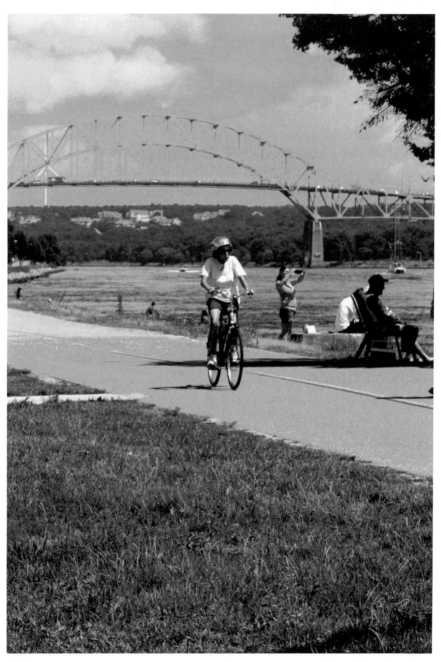

LENGTH: 13.5 miles, in 2 separate sections
SURFACE: paved
TERRAIN: flat

The Cape Cod Canal's two waterfront bike paths are free of road intersections, cooled by almost everpresent breezes, and entertained by a variety of boats plying the channel.

RULES & SAFETY:
- Bicyclists should yield to pedestrians.
- Keep to the right, pass on the left, and alert others (*"On your left..."*) when approaching from behind.
- Be especially cautious when children or pets are present since their movements can be unpredictable.
- Step off the trail when stopped so others can pass.
- Note that broken shells, dropped onto the bike path by birds, can be a hazard to bicycle tires.
- Swimming is prohibited in the canal.
- Pets must be leashed and their wastes removed.
- The area is open only during daylight hours.
- Staff patrol regularly to assist visitors and enforce these rules. Service vehicles sometimes use the bike paths.

ORIENTATION:
The bike paths follow each side of the canal and do not connect. Linking the two sides is not recommended as it requires the use of sidewalks on the Bourne and Sagamore bridges which are busy with traffic.

Note that wind can have a noticeable effect along the canal and typically comes from the west. When it's blowing hard, try to plan a ride that starts heading into the wind so that the return trip will be in the easier, downwind direction.

No streets intersect the bike paths so access is confined to the trailheads shown on the map. Most trailheads provide toilets and drinking water during the warm season. Mileage is painted on the pavement at half-mile intervals to assist visitors in tracking their progress and benches are stationed at numerous points.

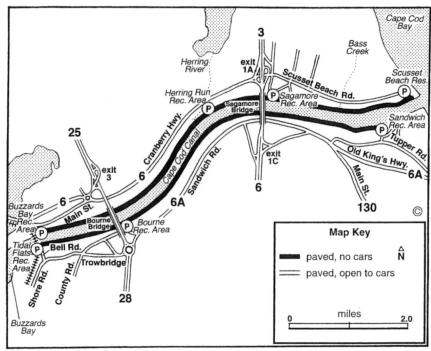

TRAIL DESCRIPTION:

The North Bikeway extends for 7 miles along the north bank of the canal. Starting from the **Buzzards Bay Recreation Area** at the western end, the trail heads eastward on a mile-long straightaway leading under the **Bourne Bridge** (1.2 miles) and curves left with the canal as it cuts through higher elevations of the Cape's interior. The bike path reaches its midpoint at the **Herring Run Recreation Area** (3.5 miles) where trailhead parking, toilets, and picnic tables enjoy a view over the waterway. Curving back to the right, the trail follows the canal under the **Sagamore Bridge** (4.5 miles), passes the fishing pier, and intersects a side trail linking nearby **Scusset Beach Reservation**. The trail ends with an excellent view from a stone pier at the canal's entrance to **Cape Cod Bay**.

The South Bikeway measures 6.6 miles long on the opposite shore. Beginning at the **Sandwich Recreation Area**, the trail enjoys a view of Cape Cod Bay before venturing westward along the south bank of the canal, curving past a power station and then following a straight line to the **Sagamore Bridge** (2 miles). A slope rises beside the trail as the canal bends left on a long, gradual turn toward its midpoint where the **Bourne Bridge** comes into view. After curving back to the right, it passes under the Bourne Bridge (5.3 miles) at a trailhead parking lot and joins the side of railroad tracks for a short distance. Look for the Aptucxet Trading Post Museum (6.2 miles), open during the warm season with information on the Pilgrims' first commercial enterprise, along with shade trees and picnic tables along this stretch. Natural surroundings enhance the last part of the trail before it ends at the **Tidal Flats Recreation Area** near the railroad bridge (6.6 miles).

BACKGROUND:

The canal was constructed between 1909 and 1914 to save ships from traveling the 135 miles around Cape Cod. It was enlarged during the 1930's by the U.S. Army Corps of Engineers when the Bourne Bridge and Sagamore Bridge were also built.

The Corps continues to manage and maintain the channel and promotes certain recreational activities. Originally intended to be service roads for the canal, these paved routes became available to bicyclists and others in the mid-1970's when interest in recreation began to grow. The Cape Cod Canal Visitor Center is located near the Sandwich Recreation Area with additional information.

DRIVING DIRECTIONS:

• **North Side:** To reach the railroad bridge parking lot from Rte. 25 in Bourne, take Exit 3 to the rotary and then follow signs for Main St. and Buzzard's Bay. The parking lot is 1 mile ahead on Main St. on the left, before a traffic signal.

• **South Side:** To reach the Sandwich Recreation Area from Rte. 6 at the Sagamore Bridge, exit at Sandwich Rd. if eastbound or Rte. 6A if westbound. Follow Sandwich Rd./Rte. 6A east, turn left on Tupper Rd. (just after Rte. 130 forks right) and continue for 1 mile, then turn left on Freezer Rd. and continue straight to the end to reach the trailhead.

TOILETS:

available at most trailhead parking lots

ADDITIONAL INFORMATION:

U.S. Army Corps of Engineers, C. C. Canal Rec.: (508) 759-5991

63 Shining Sea Bikeway
Falmouth

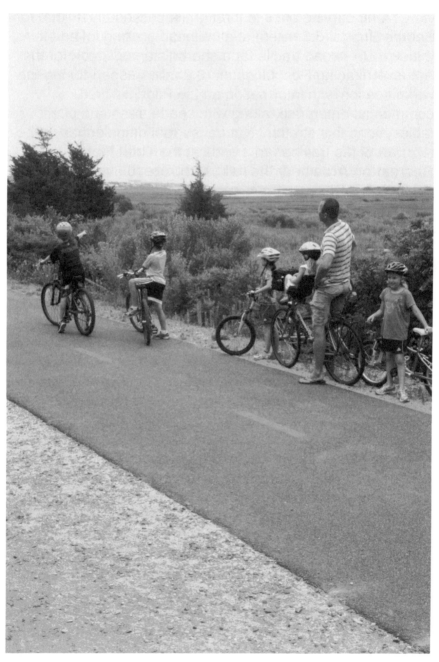

LENGTH: 10.7 miles, including 0.6-mile bike lane
SURFACE: paved
TERRAIN: slight slopes

One of the state's first rail-trails, this ride is unique for its beachfront view and great saltmarsh scenery. The 4-village route connects N. Falmouth with Woods Hole's ferry terminal, making it as convenient for locals as it is for tourists.

RULES & SAFETY:

- Bicyclists should yield to pedestrians.
- Keep to the right, pass on the left, and alert others (*"On your left..."*) when approaching from behind.
- Be especially cautious in the presence of children and pets since their movements can be unpredictable.
- Groups should ride single file.
- Step off the trail when stopped so others can pass.
- Stop at road intersections and remember that drivers might not be aware of your presence.
- Pets must be leashed and their wastes removed.

ORIENTATION:

The trail holds good scenery along its entire length with the highlights being wide vistas at Great Sippewissett Marsh and Quissett Beach. Note that these locations can also be exposed to wind and weather. In summer, the distance between Falmouth center and Woods Hole is often busy so use caution, especially near the beach.

Street signs identify road intersections and mileage markers originate from the Woods Hole ferry.

TRAIL DESCRIPTION:

Beginning at the **N. Falmouth** trailhead, find the rail-trail across **County Rd./Rte. 151** heading south beside railroad tracks (separated by fencing). The railroad curves left after a quarter-mile and the trail continues straight on a slight downslope past residential neighborhoods and woods as it intersects **Winslow Rd.** (0.6 miles), passes under **Curley Blvd.** (1.0 mile), and crosses **Wing Rd.** (1.4 miles). After traversing a cranberry bog, it reaches a cluster of

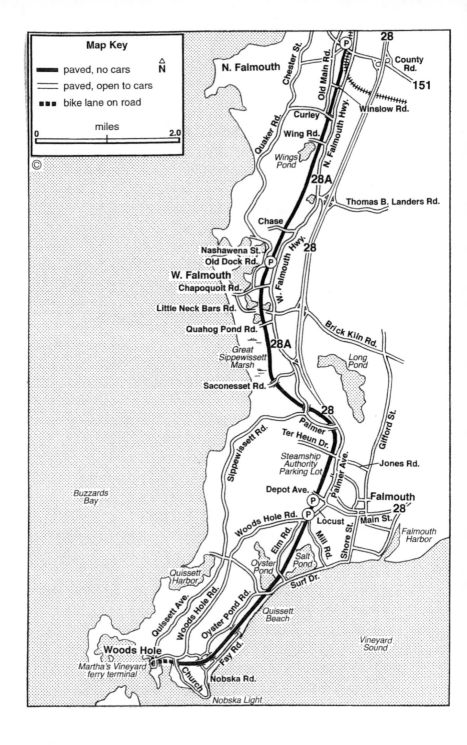

Map Key

paved, no cars

paved, open to cars

bike lane on road

N

miles

0   2.0

©

N. Falmouth

Chester St.

Old Main Rd.

N. Falmouth Hwy.

28

County Rd.

151

Winslow Rd.

Curley

Wing Rd.

Wings Pond

28A

Thomas B. Landers Rd.

Chase

W. Falmouth Hwy.

28

Nashawena St.

Old Dock Rd.

W. Falmouth

Chapoquoit Rd.

Little Neck Bars Rd.

Quahog Pond Rd.

Brick Kiln Rd.

28A

Long Pond

Great Sippewissett Marsh

Saconesset Rd.

28

Palmer

Ter Heun Dr.

Sippewissett Rd.

Gifford St.

Steamship Authority Parking Lot

Palmer Ave.

Jones Rd.

Buzzards Bay

Depot Ave.

Falmouth

28

Woods Hole Rd.

Locust

Main St.

Falmouth Harbor

Elm Rd.

Oyster Pond

Salt Pond

Mill Rd.

Shore St.

Quissett Harbor

Surf Dr.

Quissett Ave.

Woods Hole Rd.

Oyster Pond Rd.

Quissett Beach

Vineyard Sound

Woods Hole

Fay Rd.

Martha's Vineyard ferry terminal

Church

Nobska Rd.

Nobska Light

intersections at **W. Falmouth** including **Chase Rd.** (2.7 miles), **Old Dock Rd.** (3.3 miles), and **Chapoquoit Rd.** (3.6 miles). The trail continues past several ponds and then gains a broad view across **Great Sippewissett Marsh** (4.2 miles) to **Buzzards Bay**.

Returning to woods, the bike path turns southeast and rises to higher ground where a cut allows it to pass under **Saconesset Rd.** (5.1 miles) and **Palmer Ave.** (5.6 miles and again at 6.1 miles). It then curves back to the south near Rte. 28 at the outskirts of Falmouth Village crossing **Ter Heun Dr.** (6.5 miles), a **Steamship Authority parking lot**, and **Depot Ave.** (7.1 miles) at a trailhead and former station.

The trail intersects **Rte. 28** (7.5 miles) at a crosswalk (use caution) and enters quieter, natural surroundings which include a view of **Salt Pond** (8.0 miles) on the left. After intersecting **Elm Rd.** (8.5 miles) it joins a barrier beach along **Vineyard Sound**, crossing **Surf Dr.** (8.7 miles) and following the sandy shore of **Quissett Beach** for a half-mile. Watch for foot traffic crossing the trail to access the beach.

Rising back into tree-cover, the last leg has bridges over **Fay Rd.** (9.4 miles) and **Nobska Rd.** (9.8 miles) and then curves westward to reach another Steamship Authority parking lot (10.1 miles) where a 0.6-mile painted bike lane continues to the **ferry terminal** (10.7 miles) at **Woods Hole**.

BACKGROUND:

Train service along this route began in 1872 and ended in 1965. The trail originated in 1975 and was named to honor Falmouth native Katherine Lee Bates (1859-1929), author of the poem *America the Beautiful*. The trail was extended to N. Falmouth in 2009.

DRIVING DIRECTIONS:

• **Rte. 151 trailhead:** From the Bourne Bridge, follow Rte. 28 south for 6.5 miles to Rte. 151. Drive west for a half-mile to the trailhead on the right, just after railroad tracks.

• **Depot Rd. trailhead:** From the Bourne Bridge, follow Rte. 28 south for 13.4 miles, turn right on Depot Rd., then turn left at the trailhead just past the trail crossing.

TOILETS:

ferry terminal at Woods Hole, portables at some trailheads in season

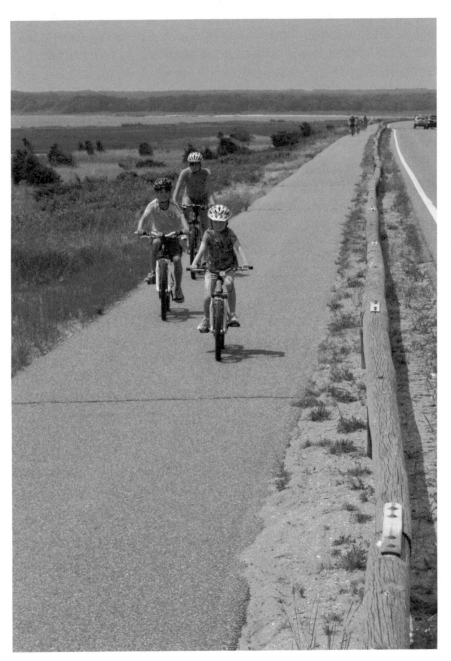

LENGTH: 31 miles
SURFACE: paved
TERRAIN: mostly flat, some slopes

Self-propelled vacationers make good use of the Vineyard's extensive network of roadside bike paths which links most of the commercial centers and tourist hot spots with enjoyable riding.

RULES & SAFETY:
- Bicyclists should yield to pedestrians.
- Keep to the right, pass on the left, and alert others (*"On your left..."*) when approaching from behind.
- Be especially cautious in the presence of children and pets since their movements can be unpredictable.
- Obey stop signs at trail/road intersections and remember that drivers might not be aware of your presence.
- Step off the trail when stopped so others can pass.

ORIENTATION:
The bike paths run from the outskirts of the ferry ports of Vineyard Haven (Tisbury) and Oak Bluffs south to the island's interior and to Edgartown. Most paths parallel main roads in gentle terrain with separation of a guardrail, mowed grass, or cover of trees while a few venture away from roads into the state forest at the center of the island.

TRAIL DESCRIPTION:
The 4.9-mile **Beach Rd.** bike path, the island's most popular, covers most of the 6.5-mile distance between the gingerbread cottages of **Oak Bluffs** and the captain's homes of **Edgartown**. The path is exposed to wind but enjoys excellent views of **Nantucket Sound** for much of the way. To find it from the Steamship Authority ferry in Oak Bluffs, turn left off the dock and follow Seaview Ave. out of town along the water for 0.7 miles. The path rolls and turns until it enters the flat, open area of **State Beach** where dunes and saltwater views line both sides of the trail for 2 miles. The path enters Edgartown as it returns to the cover of trees and continues for another mile to Edgartown-Vineyard Haven Rd.

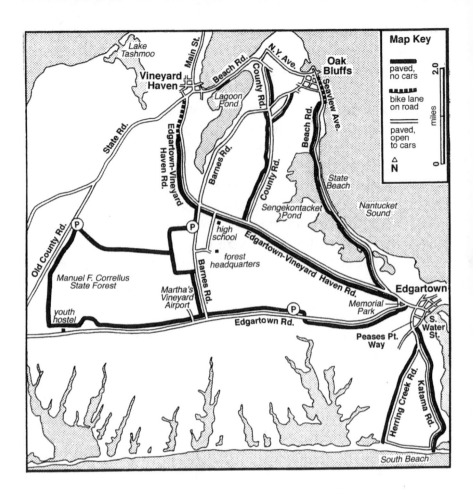

Map Key

paved,
no cars

bike lane
on road

paved,
open
to cars

N

Keep left to reach **Edgartown**, less than a mile ahead.

The 6.7-mile **Edgartown-Vineyard Haven Rd.** bike path starts at the outskirts of **Vineyard Haven**. To find it from that ferry terminal, turn left off the dock on Water St., right on Beach St., merge left at **Main St.**, then look for Edgartown-Vineyard Haven Rd. on the left. A bike lane follows the road for the first 0.6 miles until the separated path begins on the right. Rolling over small hills at first, it intersects Airport Rd. and follows a flat, straight line for most of the way to **Memorial Park** in Edgartown.

The 2.5-mile **Katama Rd.** bike path links Edgartown with a mostly flat ride to **South Beach**. Continue past Memorial Park's stacked cannon balls on Main St. for 0.2

miles and turn right on **Peases Point Way** for a quarter-mile, left on High St. to the end, right on **S. Water St.** to the end, then left on Katama Rd. A 2.1-mile path along **Herring Creek Rd.** also links South Beach for a return-trip variation.

The **Edgartown Rd.** bike path begins near Memorial Park in Edgartown heading west to the island's interior. Starting in a residential area, it passes farm fields and then woods, crossing to the north side of the road after 2.5 miles before reaching **Manuel F. Corellus State Forest** at a trailhead parking lot. The trail continues for another 1.7 miles to **Barnes Rd.** where a 10-mile loop explores the state forest west of **Martha's Vineyard Airport**. Turning right (north) on the path beside Barnes Rd., ride for a mile to the end of the airport's clearing and then around a left turn away from the road. Turn left (west) at the next intersection on a woodsy, 2.2-mile bike path to **Old County Rd.**, then keep left (south) on the path alongside that road. After a mile it veers off the road and along a field at the state forest boundary for 1.3 miles, then turns left (east) beside Edgartown Rd. in Tisbury for the 3.5-mile return leg.

BACKGROUND:

The Vineyard has been a bicycle-friendly place ever since the two-wheeled contraptions first landed on the island in the late 1800's, and Oak Bluff has the distinction of having hosted the country's first bicycle race in 1887. As an annual tide of tourists subsequently filled the island's roads, separated bike paths were conceived to ease traffic and provide recreation. The first segments were constructed in 1973 and the network has steadily expanded and improved since that time.

DRIVING DIRECTIONS:

Steamship Authority ferries link Woods Hole in Falmouth with both Vineyard Haven and Oak Bluffs. Other passenger-only ferries connect Falmouth Harbor to Oak Bluffs and Edgartown.

Trailhead parking is provided at several locations in Manuel F. Corellus State Forest at the center of the island.

TOILETS:

Vineyard Haven and Oak Bluffs ferry terminals, Edgartown bus station/visitor center on Church St.

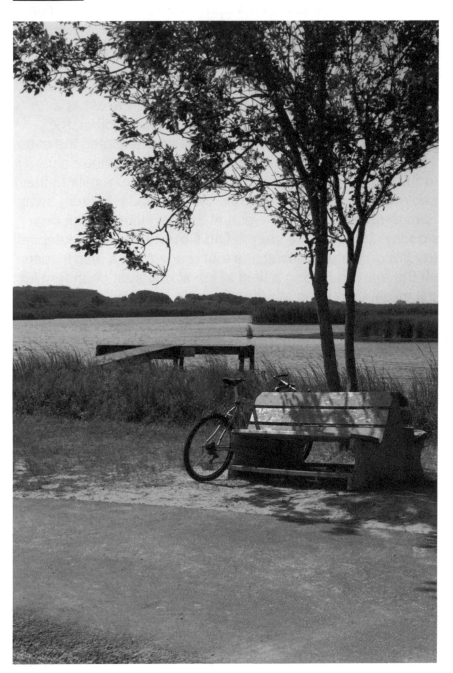

LENGTH: 32 miles
SURFACE: paved
TERRAIN: gently rolling

Extending in all directions, Nantucket's roadside bike paths connect downtown to outlying villages, beaches, and conservation lands, enabling both tourists and residents to leave their cars at home.

RULES & SAFETY:
- Bicyclists should yield to pedestrians.
- Keep to the right, pass on the left, and alert others (*"On your left..."*) when approaching from behind.
- Be especially cautious in the presence of children and pets since their movements can be unpredictable.
- When riding downtown, bicyclists are reminded not to ride on sidewalks and not to travel in the wrong direction on the many one-way streets.
- Groups should ride single file.
- Step off the trail when stopped so others can pass.
- Stop at road intersections and driveways and remember that drivers might not be aware of your presence.
- Respect nearby residents by keeping noise levels low.
- Pets should be leashed and their wastes removed.

ORIENTATION:
The island's bike paths originate at the outskirts of downtown but reaching these points from the ferry terminals can be a challenge since many of the area's narrow streets are one-way and surfaced with cobble stones, making for a bumpy ride. On-road bike routes, marked by small arrows, identify the best routes from Steamboat Wharf to the outlying bike paths.

Water fountains are distributed along the bike path network and are a helpful amenity in summer since tree shade is scarce on many routes. Benches and picnic tables also await at numerous points, portable toilets are stationed at beach parking lots, and food is available during the summer season at outlying villages such as Madaket,

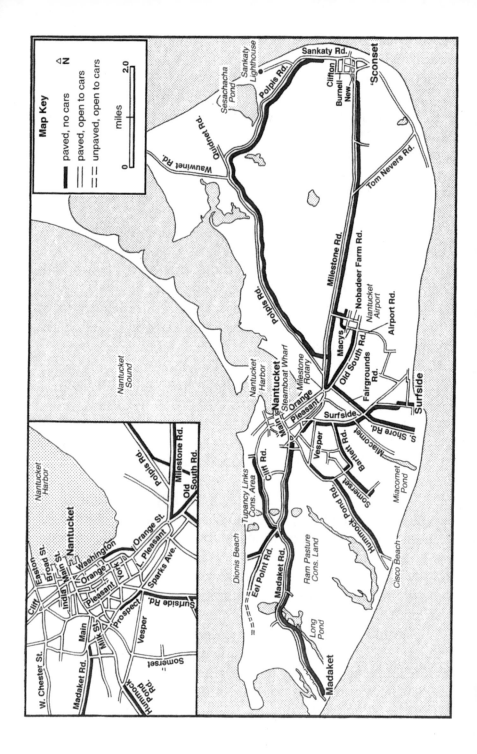

Surfside, and 'Sconset. Most bike paths are generously wide with mowed borders, stop signs, and crosswalks.

TRAIL DESCRIPTION:

The 1.7-mile **Cliff Rd.** bike path is one of the easiest to reach from **Steamboat Wharf** but also one of the hilliest. Follow Cliff Rd. uphill from the edge of town and look for the separated path beginning on the right at Sherburne Tpke. It climbs at a slight pitch to a broad field and ocean view at the **Tupancy Links Conservation Area** (0.5 miles), intersects **Eel Point Rd.** (1.6 miles) on the right where a 0.9-mile bike path leads to **Dionis Beach**, and soon ends with a sharp turn and abrupt drop to Madaket Rd.

The scenic, 5.5-mile **Madaket Rd.** bike path intersects at this point on a gently rolling route past more conservation lands to **Madaket**, a beach and cluster of homes at the island's western reach. It begins at Caton Circle where Quaker Rd., **Main St.**, and Madaket Rd. intersect. Although most of this bike path is well screened from the road, the path and road have no separation at several points including the first half-mile, so use extra caution when traffic is present. After passing a rest area at **Long Pond** (3.4 miles), the trail's approach to Madaket crosses increasing numbers of roads and driveways before it ends near the beach parking lot.

The 2.7-mile **Hummock Pond Rd.** bike path follows another scenic route heading southwest past farmland and conservation areas to **Cisco Beach**. The trail encounters slight slopes, has a buffer of trees shielding the road for part of the way, and boasts 4 water fountains along its course. Surrounding trees get progressively shorter along the second half allowing a broad, ocean view near the end.

Surfside is one of Nantucket's most popular beaches and home to the island's youth hostel. Relatively short and flat, the 2.3-mile Surfside bike path doesn't offer especially scenic views but provides easy access to the south shore's pounding waves and intersects other paths along the way. Heading south along **Surfside Rd.**, it begins at the intersection of **Vesper La.** across from the high school.

Two bike paths intersect at a four-way intersection near Surfside's midpoint. The mile-long pathway beside **South Shore Rd.** makes a straight-line route toward the ocean, interrupted by many driveways, but requires a short ride on gravel Hillside Ave. and then a hike through dunes in order to reach the beach. In the opposite direction, 0.9-mile Fairgrounds Rd. Bike Path crosses flat terrain, enjoys good separation from the road, and ends at **Old South Rd.** near the **Milestone Rotary** where more trails originate.

The 1.5-mile Old South Rd. bike path connects the rotary to **Nantucket Airport**. Rolling with small slopes, it is well-separated from the roadway but contends with numerous side street intersections near the airport. At the end, turn left on **Macy's La.** (opposite **Airport Rd.**) to reach the 0.7-mile **Nobadeer Farm Rd.** bike path which follows a woodsy route past a school and athletic fields, crosses Nobadeer Farm Rd., and continues north to **Milestone Rd.**

Sitting on a bluff above the ocean at the island's eastern tip, Siasconset (shortened to **'Sconset**) is Nantucket's most distant destination and accessible by two bike paths which combine to form a 15.5-mile loop from the rotary. The 6-mile **Milestone** bike path (also known as the 'Sconset Bike Path) closely follows the edge of Milestone Rd. from the rotary eastward to 'Sconset dipping at a few wrinkles in otherwise flat terrain. True to its name, the route has stone markers placed at 1-mile intervals which offer a helpful means of plotting progress and a welcome diversion along the road's monotonously straight course. Side by side, the road and path crest a hill near the intersection of **Tom Nevers Rd.** with a nice view of the island's cranberry bog, the **Sankaty Lighthouse**, and the village 2 miles ahead.

The 8.2-mile **Polpis Rd.** bike path is a more interesting, and longer, route to 'Sconset and starts from the Milestone Bike Path a half-mile east of the rotary and just beyond the intersection of Polpis Rd. Turning frequently and rolling with small ups and downs, this trail follows the south side of Polpis Rd. with excellent screening and separation for most of the way but intersects numerous driveways that deserve caution when crossing. The trail passes the Nantucket Shipwreck and Lifesaving Museum (2.4 miles) and offers a distant view of the Sankaty Lighthouse (6.8 miles) before ending beside **Sankaty Rd.** at the outskirts of 'Sconset. To return on the Milestone Bike Path about a mile away, continue south on Sankaty Rd. (which becomes Shell St.) to the village center, then turn right on Main St. and look for the bike path ahead on the left side.

BACKGROUND:

Named with a Native American word meaning *the land far out to sea*, Nantucket is separated by 25 miles of ocean waters and is one of Massachusetts' most unique summer retreats. Much of the island's charm originates from its whaling heritage of the late 1700's and early 1800's when the town was the capitol of the industry with a fleet of ships plying waters around the world. When whale oil gave way to petroleum fuels, the town endured a long period of decline until tourism restored prosperity.

Wise planning has preserved Nantucket. The establishment of a historic district has fostered the restoration of downtown buildings and the protection of hundreds of acres of open space has served the rest of the island well. Construction of the bike path network began in the 1970's and continues to progress, easing traffic while providing enjoyable exercise and recreation.

DRIVING DIRECTIONS:

Ferries serve Nantucket from Hyannis and Oak Bluffs; contact the ferry companies listed below for schedules and information. Visitors are encouraged to leave their cars on the mainland.

TOILETS:

visitor information center at 25 Federal St., Town Pier, Straight Wharf, Steamboat Wharf, and at public beaches

ADDITIONAL INFORMATION:

Nantucket Visitor Services & Information Bureau, 25 Federal St., www.nantucket-ma.gov/departments/visitor
Mass. Steamship Authority, www.steamshipauthority.com
Hy-Line Cruises, www.hy-linecruises.com

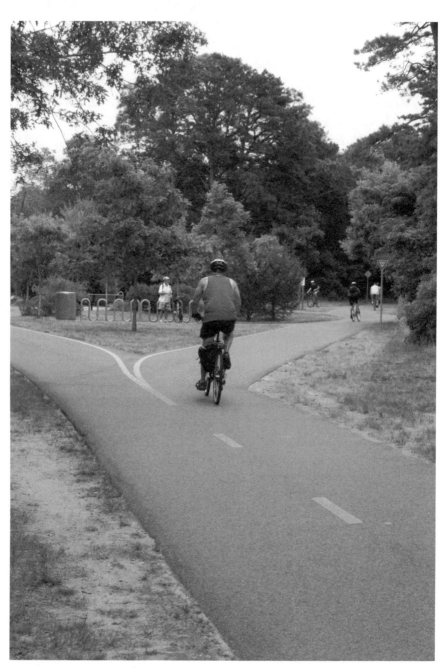

LENGTH: 26.1 miles (including 0.9 miles under construction), plus 23.4 miles of side trails nearby

SURFACE: paved

TERRAIN: gentle slopes

The granddaddy of Massachusetts rail-trails, Cape Cod's famous bike path draws a parade of self-propelled traffic past quiet woods, cranberry bogs, kettle ponds, and saltmarshes. Side trails branch with additional options.

RULES & SAFETY:

• Bicyclists should yield to pedestrians.

• Keep to the right, pass on the left, and alert others (*"On your left..."*) when approaching from behind.

• Be especially cautious in the presence of children and pets since their movements can be unpredictable.

• Groups should ride single file.

• Step off the trail when stopped so others can pass.

• Stop at road intersections and remember that drivers might not be aware of your presence.

• Respect nearby residents by keeping noise levels low.

• Pets must be leashed and their wastes removed.

• Sections of trail under construction are closed to use.

• Watch for additional information posted at trailheads.

ORIENTATION:

Numerous trailheads provide starting points. The most popular stretch is from Dennis to Orleans where riders enjoy interesting natural scenery, plenty of shade, and an array of bridges, tunnels, and even a trail rotary. North of Orleans, the rail-trail is less crowded on busy days but exposed to sun along many parts. West of Dennis, the new Yarmouth section offers additional trailhead parking but includes a 0.9-mile section at the Bass River which is temporarily closed for bridge construction until 2018.

The Cape Cod Rail-Tr. intersects significant side trails including: the 7.6-mile Old Colony Rail-Tr. from Harwich to Chatham, 8 miles of bike paths at Nickerson State Park (Chapter 67) in Brewster, and the 2-mile Nauset Bicycle Tr.

in Eastham. In addition, local bike paths branch into Dennis and Yarmouth.

Street signs at road intersections assist with plotting progress on this long trail and mileage is marked on granite posts at 1-mile intervals. Note that some intersecting streets and smaller trailside parking locations are not displayed on the accompanying map. Bike shops, ice cream stands, and other provisions await at points along the way.

TRAIL DESCRIPTION:

Starting at the **Rte. 134** trailhead in Dennis, the rail-trail extends in two directions. Heading west (left from the parking lot, the trail's newest section rises on a bridge over Rte. 134, intersects **Main St.** after a quarter-mile at another trailhead parking lot, and borders protected conservation land before reaching a bridge over the **Bass River** beside the highway noise of **Rte. 6**. Here it crosses the Yarmouth town line, enjoys a southerly view down the river, and contnues paralleling Rte. 6 to **N. Main St.** (1.8 miles).

The trail continues westward veering away from the highway into quieter surroundings as it passes a combination of woods and industrial properties along parallel Whites Path. It passes a trailhead parking lot at **Station Ave.** (3.5 miles) where another bridge carries the trail high over the road, parallels railroad tracks for a short distance, then leaves the rail line to join paved trails circling a park off **Old Town House Rd.** (4.0 miles).

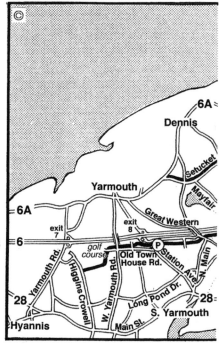

A Yarmouth bike path continues west for another 2 miles with small slopes in

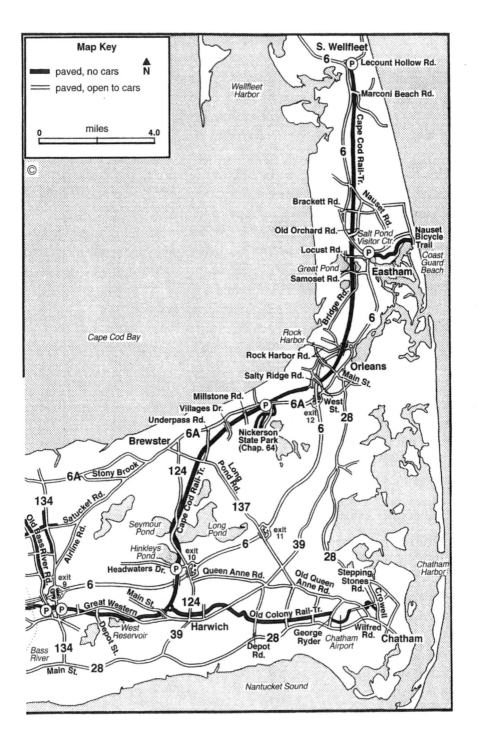

mostly wooded surroundings. It begins by skirting a recycling facility, intersects **W. Yarmouth Rd.**, passes through the Bayberry Hills **golf course**, and ends at **Higgins Crowell Rd.** Note that bicycles are restricted from using the golf course's paved cart paths.

Heading east from the Rte. 134 trailhead in Dennis, the Cape Cod Rail-Tr. stretches for 22.1 miles. The trail begins in a wooded corridor, passes an industrial area near the diagonal crossing of **Great Western Rd.** (0.7 miles), enters Harwich near **Depot Rd.** (1.3 miles), and passes a brief water view at **West Reservoir** (1.5 miles). It enters an area of cranberry bogs near a second intersection of Great Western Rd. (2.3 miles) and narrows as it passes through a tunnel under **Main St.** (3.2 miles), then emerges at a rail-trail rotary and resting area (3.3 miles).

Here the 7.6-mile **Old Colony Rail-Tr.** forks right (east) with a mostly uphill ride past **Harwich** center to the outskirts of **Chatham**. This side trail detours from the original rail line at three points, the first occuring at a missing bridge over a low area where the trail curves downhill and then climbs back to level ground. After crossing **Rte. 137** at a trailhead parking area, another detour circles the **Chatham Airport** where bicyclists turn right on **George Ryder Rd.** and ride for a quarter-mile, turn left on a paved trail along the airport's southern perimeter fence, and continue on **Wilfred Rd.** (the original rail bed) for 0.6 miles. Crossing **Queen Anne Rd.**, the trail detours again with a climb alongside **Stepping Stones Rd.** before ending at **Crowell Rd.**

Continuing on the Cape Cod Rail-Tr., riders head north from the trail rotary on a slight incline through almost a mile of woods to a bridge over **Rte. 6** (4.3 miles) and descend to the **Headwaters Dr.** trailhead (4.7 miles). It then enters a scenic area of cranberry bogs and ponds including **Hinckleys Pond** on the left, **Long Pond** on the right, and **Seymour Pond** on the left, crossing **Rte. 124** three times along the way.

Entering Brewster (6.0 miles), the trail returns to

woods and rises on a 2-mile incline to a high point at the **Long Pond Rd./Rte. 137** trailhead (8.0 miles). It gains a slight downslope to **Underpass Rd.** (8.5 miles) then flattens as it passes under Villages Dr. (9.4 miles) and intersects Millstone Rd. (10.0 miles). **Nickerson State Park** (Chapter 67) appears on the right 10.6 miles from the Dennis trailhead and offers parking, toilets, water, picnic tables, a beach, campsites, and 8 miles of hilly, paved bike paths.

Continuing northeastward, the rail-trail enters a tunnel under **Rte. 6A** and follows a shady corridor for the next mile and a half until it reaches Namskaket Creek where a saltwater marsh and view of **Cape Cod Bay** mark the Orleans town line. Ahead, it joins the end of **Salty Ridge Rd.** (12.2 miles) where a marked, on-road detour avoids a missing bridge over Rte. 6. Keep left with Salty Ridge, turn right on **West Rd.** (crossing Rte. 6), then look for the rail-trail resuming on the left at a crosswalk (12.5 miles).

The trail reaches **Orleans** center in another half-mile and crosses **Main St.** (13.2 miles) in the downtown shopping area. Returning to woods, it gradually curves north while descending a slight slope for the next 0.7 miles and then rises on another bridge over Rte. 6 (13.9 miles) and **Rock Harbor Rd.** near the Orleans rotary. Entering Eastham nearby, the rail-trail straightens along a powerline corridor for most of the remaining 8.2 miles and is exposed to greater amounts of sun for much of this distance. The next 2.7 miles stay flat as the trail crosses a marsh at Boat Meadow River, intersects several roads, and passes a cluster of ponds before reaching **Locust Rd.** (16.6 miles).

Nearby, the 2-mile **Nauset Bicycle Trail** ventures east to the Atlantic Ocean. To find it, turn right on Locust Rd. and ride for a third of a mile, turn left on **Salt Pond Rd.** and continue for a tenth of a mile, and cross Rte. 6 at a traffic signal. The bike path starts on the other side in front of the National Seashore's **Salt Pond Visitor Ctr.** and takes a rolling, curving route through small hills and cedar forest, crosses a bridge through a saltmarsh, and ends with a grand

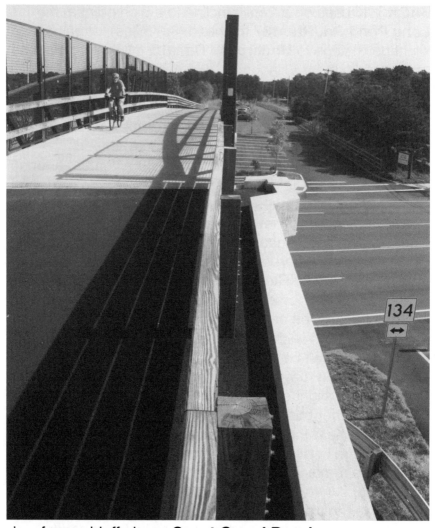

view from a bluff above **Coast Guard Beach**.

   The Cape Cod Rail-Tr. continues north from Locust Rd. for another 5.5 miles. After intersecting Kingsbury Beach Rd. (16.9 miles), it negotiates curved slopes at a tunnel under Rte. 6 (17.0 miles) and flattens in the area of **Brackett Rd.** (17.8 miles) and **Nauset Rd.** (18.5 miles). The trail encounters a few slight slopes after entering Wellfleet where it intersects **Marconi Beach Rd.** (21.2 miles) and enjoys a westward view over **Wellfleet Harbor** before ending at **Lecount Hollow Rd.** (22.1 miles).

BACKGROUND:

The Cape Cod Central Railroad created this route in the mid-1800's as tourists discovered the region. Rails were extended eastward in phases reaching Orleans in 1865, Wellfleet in 1870, and Chatham in 1887. After the Bourne and Sagamore bridges were completed in 1935, automobiles crippled the railroad's passenger service but freight trains continued to use the line until the mid-1960's. The state acquired the route in 1978 and the first section of rail-trail was opened from Dennis to Eastham in 1981. Since then the bike path was extended north to S. Wellfleet in 1995 and west to Yarmouth in 2017, and the Old Colony branch was developed east to Chatham in 2007. Future plans call for trail construction west toward Hyannis with the hope that the trail will eventually connect Falmouth (Chap. 63) and Provincetown (Chap. 68).

DRIVING DIRECTIONS:

• **Yarmouth trailhead:** From Rte. 6 take exit 8, follow Station Ave. south for 0.4 miles, and park in the lot on the left just after the trail overpass.

• **Dennis trailhead:** From Rte. 6 take exit 9 for Rte. 134 south and find the trailhead on the left after a half-mile. For additional parking continue south on Rte. 134 to the next traffic signal, turn right on Upper County Rd., right on Main St., and look for the Cape Cod Rail-Tr. sign on the left.

• **Harwich trailhead:** From Rte. 6 take exit 10 and follow Rte. 124 north. Turn left on Headwaters Dr. and continue for a third of a mile to the parking lot on the left.

• **Brewster trailhead:** From Rte. 6 take exit 12 and follow Rte. 6A west for 1.6 miles. Turn left at the entrance to Nickerson State Park and park in the lot on the right.

• **Salt Pond Visitor Center:** From Rte. 6 (2.8 miles east of the Orleans rotary) turn right on Doane Rd., then immediately right at the parking lot.

• **Wellfleet trailhead:** From Rte. 6 (8.3 miles east of the Orleans rotary) turn right on Lecount Hollow Rd. and look for the trailhead parking a short ahead on the right.

TOILETS:

Nickerson State Park (Brewster), Salt Pond Visitor Ctr. (Eastham), seasonally at other locations

ADDITIONAL INFORMATION:

Nickerson State Park, Brewster, (508) 896-4615

67 Nickerson State Park

Brewster

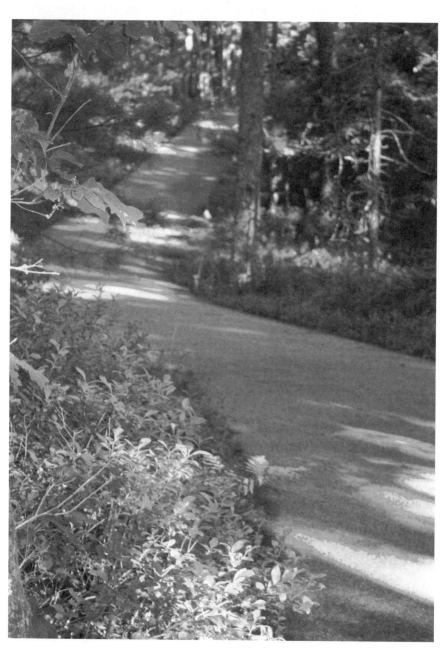

LENGTH: 8 miles
SURFACE: paved
TERRAIN: hilly

Nickerson's vast woodlands hold a hillier, curvier, and quieter alternative to the adjoining Cape Cod Rail-Trail. Winding through trees, this rolling ride is a complement to the park's campgrounds and freshwater ponds.

RULES & SAFETY:
- Bicyclists should yield to pedestrians.
- Some trails have big slopes, sharp curves, relatively narrow widths, and two-way traffic so ride at a safe speed and stay alert for on-coming bicyclists.
- Keep to the right, pass on the left, and alert others (*"On your left..."*) when approaching from behind.
- Use extra caution when children and pets are present since their movements can be unpredictable.
- Watch for cracks and bumps in the paved surface and areas of accummulated leaves and pine needles which can be slippery, especially when wet.
- Stop at road crossings and assume that drivers do not see you.
- Do not block gates when parking since work crews and emergency vehicles always need access.
- Swimming is permitted only at designated locations which are staffed during the summer season.

ORIENTATION:
The bike paths extend southward from the main trailhead at the Cape Cod Rail-Trail (Chapter 66) on Rte. 6A, and branch in loops at several points to allow return trip variations. Trail maps are provided at a few locations and trail names are labeled at intersections along with directions back to the main trailhead. The small number of road crossings, made apparent by metal gates blocking vehicle entry, provide additional landmarks in otherwise unbroken forest. Note that the highest elevation is at the center of the park near the midpoint of the trail network.

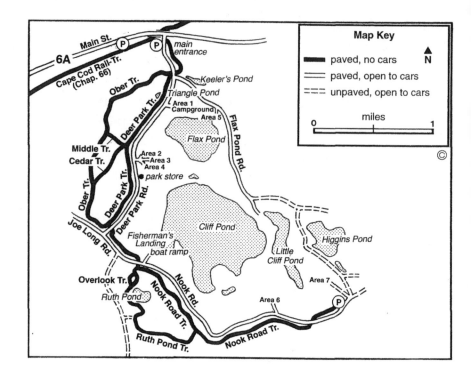

TRAIL DESCRIPTIONS:

Begin at Nickerson's **main entrance** beside **Rte. 6A**
where a trailhead parking lot offers picnic tables, toilets, and
information near the **Cape Cod Rail-Trail** (Chapter 66). The
1.4-mile **Deer Park Tr.** begins on the opposide (east) side of
Deer Park Rd., the park's entrance drive, and rises on a
slope through woods. After passing under powerlines, it
crosses Deer Park Rd. (0.4 miles), forks left at the **Ober Tr.**,
and climbs two strenuous hills along the next half-mile to an
intersection with **Middle Tr.** and **Cedar Tr.** (0.9 miles). Deer
Park Tr. climbs another uphill to its high point near the **park
store** then flattens for a half-mile before ending at a second
intersection of the Ober Tr. and Deer Park Rd. (1.4 miles).

The 1.6-mile **Ober Tr.** turns right at this point and
follows the park boundary north back toward the trailhead. It
begins with a long downslope beside **Joe Long Rd.**, rolls
and turns through woods to intersect both Cedar Tr. and
Middle Tr., then hits bigger slopes before ending at Deer

Park Tr. and Deer Park Rd. The 0.5-mile **Cedar Tr.** follows the edge of a cedar swamp for most of the way back to Deer Park Tr. and intersects the shorter **Middle Tr.** which also connects the Ober. Combining Deer Park Tr., Ober Tr., and Cedar Tr. completes a 3.1-mile ride from the trailhead.

Nook Road Tr. extends from the south end of Deer Park Tr. into more challenging terrain. Dropping on a big slope, it crosses **Nook Rd.** near **Fisherman's Landing** at **Cliff Pond**, forks left at the Ruth Pond Tr. (0.5 miles), and then climbs through a stand of white pines. After passing the south end of Ruth Pond Tr. (1.1 miles), it contends with several steep slopes, flattens opposite the **Area 6 Campground**, and drops to a final crossing of Nook Rd. (2.0 miles). The trail rolls with small slopes before dead-ending at a parking area (2.3 miles) near the **Area 7 Campground**, 3.7 miles from the park's main entrance.

The 1.3-mile **Ruth Pond Tr.** is a worthwhile return trip variation circling pristine **Ruth Pond**. It curves through woods in a terrain of small hills with views of the pond through trees near the midpoint. The **Overlook Tr.** offers another side trip over a small hill.

BACKGROUND:

Nickerson State Park was established in 1934 by a gift of land from the Nickerson family of Brewster. The 1900-acre park, Cape Cod's largest, was developed by the Civilian Conservation Corps during the 1930's when roads and campgrounds were built.

The paved bike paths were constructed in the 1970's in response to growing interest in recreation and fitness and to complement the park's 420 campsites and public swimming beach. Surrounding these facilities, Nickerson's quiet forests and freshwater ponds are a contrast to the Cape's other attractions.

DRIVING DIRECTIONS:

From Rte. 6 take Exit 12 and follow Rte. 6A west toward Brewster for 1.5 miles. Turn left at the park's main entrance and park in the lot on the right.

TOILETS:

trailhead parking lot at the main entrance

ADDITIONAL INFORMATION:

Nickerson State Park, (508) 896-3491

68 Province Lands Bicycle Trail
Provincetown

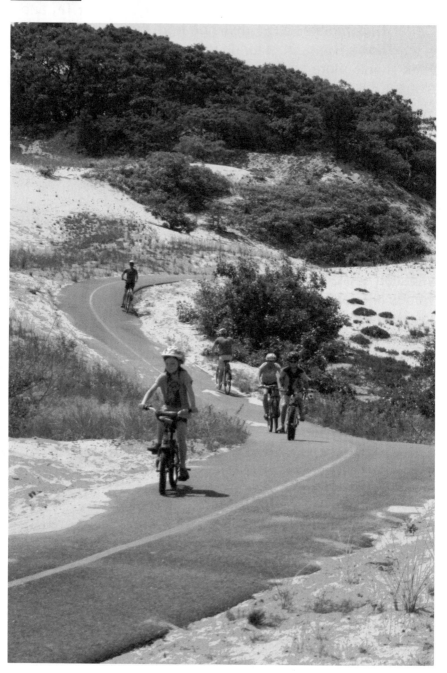

LENGTH: 7.5 miles, including 5.5-mile loop
SURFACE: paved
TERRAIN: hilly

The state's most spectacular bike path is a lively loop in a unique landscape of mountainous sand dunes, shady forests, and ocean beaches at the tip of Cape Cod.

RULES & SAFETY:
· Bicyclists should yield to pedestrians.
· The trail has abrupt hills, sharp corners, and two-way traffic so keep to the right side, ride at a safe speed, and use care when passing.
· Use extra caution in the presence of children since their movements can be unpredictable.
· Step off the trail when stopped to allow others to pass.
· Watch for sand that has accumulated on the trail, which makes turning and braking more dangerous.
· Bicycling is not permitted off the paved trails. Respect the fragile environment of the surrounding dunes.
· In-line skating is not permitted on the trail.
· Pets are not allowed.

ORIENTATION:
The trail includes a 5.5-mile loop plus 5 branches leading to outlying locations. Signs give directions to destinations and warn of curves, slopes, and intersections.

Four parking lots, each with toilets, provide access to the trail although two are used primarily for beach access. The best trailheads for bicyclists are the Beech Forest parking lot which is located at a low elevation and provides direct access to the flattest portion of the trail, and the popular Province Lands Visitor Center parking lot which also serves an interpretive museum with a panoramic view from its high elevation. Remember that starting your ride from a high point will require ending with a hill climb.

TRAIL DESCRIPTION:
Beginning at the **Beech Forest** trailhead, turn right on the paved trail to follow the loop in the clockwise direction.

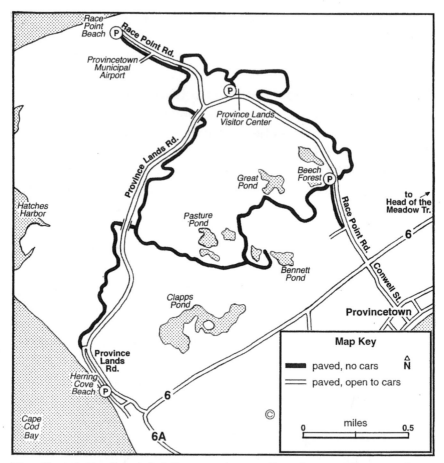

The first 1.5 miles of riding explore a flat, forested area of wetlands and small ponds and intersect a side trail to **Bennett Pond** on the left. The surroundings change dramatically beyond **Pasture Pond** where the trail climbs a long hill and leaves the forest shade for open dunes, cresting the slope with a distant view before descending in zig-zags to a trail intersection (2.0 miles).

Here a mile-long spur on the left leads southwest to **Herring Cove Beach** with some of the bike path's biggest slopes and most intriguing scenery of sand and dunes. The trail utilizes a tunnel under **Province Lands Rd.** and parallels the road for part of the way.

Continuing on the main loop, the trail turns north with flat terrain at first, then climbs several uphills in broad switchbacks and descends sharply to a second tunnel under Province Lands Rd. (3.0 miles). After another uphill it reaches **Race Point Rd.** (3.6 miles) where a flat, 0.4-mile spur intersects on the left and leads to **Race Point Beach**, passing **Provincetown Municipal Airport** along the way.

Cross Race Point Rd. to continue on the loop. After a 0.4-mile uphill, another spur leads to the **Province Lands Visitor Center** (4.0 miles) on the right while the main loop continues upward through a stand of twisted, stunted pitch pines. Stop to enjoy the impressive ocean view at the top before descending into the shade of oaks on the other side. At the bottom, the trail turns through flatter terrain paralleling Race Point Rd. for another mile, then crosses the road to return to the Beech Forest trailhead (5.5 miles). Another spur trail forks left at this point and continues beside Race Point Road for a quarter-mile toward Provincetown.

Nearby in Truro, The National Seashore's less used, 1.9-mile **Head of the Meadow Bicycle Tr.** is a short drive away. This flat, paved, point-to-point trail parallels the ocean shoreline but is concealed from the water as it follows the edge of a salt meadow between the ends of High Head Rd. and Head of the Meadow Rd. off Rte. 6.

BACKGROUND:

Part of the Cape Cod National Seashore, the Province Lands Bicycle Trail was created by the National Park Service in the 1970's to provide both a recreational resource and a means of appreciating the area's unique expanse of huge dunes, inland forests and ponds, and high ocean viewpoints.

DRIVING DIRECTIONS:

Traveling Rte. 6 east toward Provincetown, turn right on Race Point Rd. following signs to the Province Lands Visitor Center. Park at either the Beech Forest trailhead located 0.5 miles ahead on the left or the Province Lands Visitor Center trailhead located 1.5 miles ahead on the right.

TOILETS:

Beech Forest, Province Lands Visitor Center, Herring Cove, and Race Point.

ADDITIONAL INFORMATION:

Cape Cod National Seashore, www.nps.gov/caco

Appendix
List of Organizations

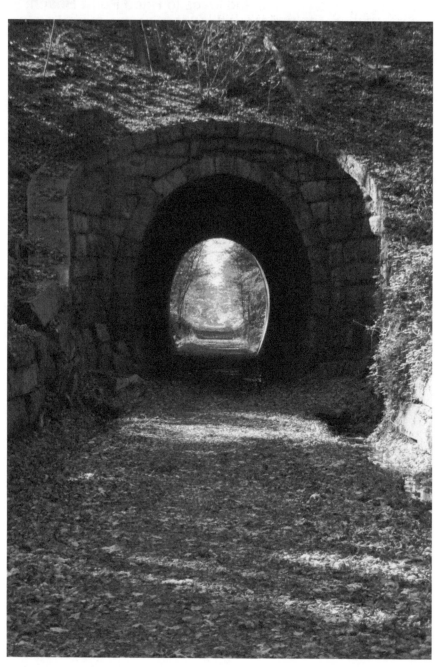

Bay Circuit Alliance, baycircuit.org

Biking and Walking Alliance, peoplepoweredmovement.org

Boston Dept. of Parks & Recreation,
boston.gov/departments/parks-and-recreation

East Coast Greenway Alliance, greenway.org

League of American Bicyclists, bikeleague.org

Massachusetts Assn. of Regional Planning Agencies,
massmarpa.org

Massachusetts Bay Transit Authority, mbta.com

Massachusetts Bicycle Coalition, massbike.org

Massachusetts Dept. of Conservation & Recreation,
mass.gov/dcr

Massachusetts Dept. of Fish & Game,
mass.gov/orgs/department-of-fish-and-game

Massachusetts Dept. of Transportation, Highway Division,
mass.gov/orgs/highway-division

Metropolitan Area Planning Council, mapc.org

New England Mountain Biking Association, nemba.org

Rails-to-Trails Conservancy, railstotrails.org

PeopleForBikes, peopleforbikes.org

The Trust for Public Land, tpl.org

The Trustees of Reservations, thetrustees.org

walkBoston, walkboston.org

Rules of the Bike Path:

1. Keep to the right.

2. Pass on the left after audibly signaling.

3. Yield to pedestrians.

4. Stop at road intersections.

5. Be alert.

6. Do not obstruct traffic.